CRAM SESSION IN

Evaluation of Sports Concussion

A Handbook for Students & Clinicians

CRAM SESSION IN
Evaluation of Sports Concussion
A Handbook for Students & Clinicians

TAMERAH N. HUNT, PHD, AT

Assistant Professor
The Ohio State University
Athletic Training Division
College of Medicine
School of Health & Rehabilitation Sciences
Columbus, Ohio

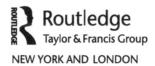

Routledge
Taylor & Francis Group

NEW YORK AND LONDON

Dr. Tamerah N. Hunt has no financial or proprietary interest in the materials presented herein.

First published in 2013 by SLACK Incorporated

Published in 2024 by Routledge
605 Third Avenue, New York, NY 10158

and by Routledge
4 Park Square, Milton Park, Abingdon, Oxon, OX14 4RN

Routledge is an imprint of the Taylor & Francis Group, an informa business

Library of Congress Cataloging-in-Publication Data

Hunt, Tamerah N.
Cram session in evaluation of sports concussion : a handbook for students & clinicians / Tamerah N. Hunt.
p. ; cm.
Includes bibliographical references and index.
ISBN 9781617110665 (alk. paper)
I. Title.
[DNLM: 1. Brain Concussion--Handbooks. 2. Athletic Injuries--Handbooks.
WL 39]
617.1'027--dc23
2012046133

ISBN: 9781617110665 (pbk)
ISBN: 9781003523376 (ebk)

DOI: 10.4324/9781003523376

Dedication

This book is dedicated to my family—

My mother and father, who inspired me to reach for my dreams while holding me accountable for the work it takes to achieve them.

My sister and brother-in-law, who consistently remind me to relax, have fun, and enjoy life.

Lastly, my nephews Alan and Sean, who are constant reminders of why I work so hard to make athletics safe for the future.

Contents

Dedication v

Acknowledgments ix

About the Author xi

Preface xiii

Foreword by Kevin M. Guskiewicz, PhD, ATC xv

Introduction xvii

Chapter 1   Introduction 1

Chapter 2   Differential Diagnoses 19

Chapter 3   Concussion Evaluation Assessments
                and Clinical Tools 35

Chapter 4   Management and Recovery of
                Sport-Related Concussion 77

Chapter 5   Return to Participation Guidelines 93

Chapter 6   Return to School/Work Accommodations 99

Chapter 7   Legal Precedent and Cases 107

Chapter 8   Prevention 119

Suggested Readings 127

Index 131

Acknowledgments

I would like to take a moment to acknowledge all who have supported me while I worked on this project. To my friends, colleagues, and students— I cannot tell you how much I appreciate your encouragement, patience, and support as I worked to finish this book. I would also like to thank Dr. Michael Ferrara, Dr. Jeffrey Konin, Dr. Thomas Best, and Darryl Conway for their mentorship and support. I could not have done this without you.

I would also like to acknowledge the Columbus City, Prince Georges, Jackson, and Richland County student-athletes for reminding me of the importance of medical care in their school systems. Thank you for cooperating with testing and for providing first-hand experience with concussion evaluation at the high school level.

I would like to especially acknowledge the Columbus City School Traumatic Brain Injury team, specifically Sara Timms, for her advanced knowledge and hard work to return the student-athlete, not just the athlete.

Lastly, I would like to thank Brien Cummings and Stephanie Wieland from SLACK Incorporated for their support, hard work, and diligence, as well as for helping me to maintain my sanity through this writing process.

About the Author

Tamerah N. Hunt, PhD, AT, received her undergraduate degree in athletic training from the University of Delaware. She received her master of science degree at James Madison University and continued to the University of Georgia where she received her doctorate in kinesiology. Following completion of her doctoral work, Dr. Hunt became an assistant professor at the University of South Carolina, teaching in the undergraduate and graduate athletic training programs. Dr. Hunt currently works at The Ohio State University (OSU) as the Director of Research for the OSU Sports Concussion Program and as Assistant Professor of Health and Rehabilitation Sciences.

Dr. Hunt was a high school athletic trainer for 4 years, during which she obtained first-hand experience with concussions and realized the lack of information available for allied health care professionals working in high schools. Her interest in this often medically neglected population triggered her research of concussions in high school athletes.

As a researcher, Dr. Hunt focuses on youth concussion assessment and has worked with high school districts in Ohio, South Carolina, Georgia, and Maryland. Dr. Hunt examines high school recovery patterns, effort given to concussion assessment, comorbidities associated with concussion, and the educational intervention tools used in multiple populations. This research has led to grant funding to examine concussion in high school athletics.

Dr. Hunt is a former National Athletic Trainers' Association Research and Education Foundation Postgraduate Scholarship recipient. She has authored various articles on concussion, youth injuries, and grade inflation and has given numerous regional, national, and international presentations as a guest speaker and clinician.

Preface

This book began as a tribute to my students. When teaching sophomore-level students head, neck, and spine evaluation, something dawned on me. The difficulty in understanding concussion evaluation was not in understanding the injury itself; it was in understanding the basis of evaluation and the tools that were available. I looked further into the clinical evaluation and management of concussion and found that more experienced athletic trainers were not fully aware of the tools that were available during the evaluation process or for returning athletes to school and work. Working alongside a local school district's traumatic brain injury team, we developed a clinical paradigm that was so helpful for these student-athletes that I wanted to share it. Within this team I learned so much regarding the special accommodations available that could be used across multiple settings. While we accept that concussive injuries occur in any sport and at any time, having a thorough understanding of the injury, differential diagnoses, assessment, and management plan for concussion will provide the best quality of care for anyone with a concussive injury.

This book is designed as a reference for any clinician, experienced or new, who works with concussed athletes. Written to focus on the evaluation process of concussion, it includes new clinical techniques, laws, and management tools to help develop safe and efficient evaluations and clinical practices for athletics.

Tamerah N. Hunt, PhD, AT

Foreword

Cram Session in Evaluation of Sports Concussion: A Handbook for Students & Clinicians by Tamerah N. Hunt, PhD, AT, is a unique and interesting monograph that will become a valuable resource for clinicians involved in the management of sports concussion. The breadth of information covered by Dr. Hunt is quite impressive and makes for easy reading. It is far from a "cram" session because the book is rather comprehensive, but it is indexed in a way that allows it to serve as an effective instruction guide to concussion management. Readers are provided with a historical perspective of how concussion research has evolved and is leading to many of the best practice guidelines developed by various sports medicine associations and sport organizing bodies. Yet, Dr. Hunt illustrates that sometimes standard guidelines or protocols cannot be applied because these injuries can present in different ways and ultimately recover in an atypical manner.

Like many chapters or books on concussion, *Cram Session in Evaluation of Sports Concussion* covers the standard definitions and pathophysiology of concussion and more serious traumatic brain injuries such as subdural and epidural hematomas and second impact syndrome. But, this book is different in that it provides user-friendly algorithms such as a "concussion concept map" to help clinicians triage the injury and work through the assessment to reach a diagnosis through a systematic approach. The additional topical areas on return to school/work accommodations and on developing and implementing a concussion management plan make this book especially unique. Dr. Hunt provides examples of concussion policies, concussion education tools, and Web sites with recommendations and policies for managing concussion.

I have often said that concussions are like snowflakes, as no two are alike. Therefore, no cookbook or calendar can specify exactly how they should be managed. Clinicians need to have all their resources available to work through the challenges of managing an injury that has often been described as a hidden or invisible injury. We must counsel our athletes about the short- and long-term risks of not reporting symptoms, returning to play while still experiencing symptoms, or not modifying risky behaviors that can predispose athletes to future concussions. This book can serve as a guide in that respect. No checkbox system can be applied to every concussion, and because concussions are diverse and unique injuries that affect each athlete differently, we must learn how to treat them individually. Likewise, concussed athletes are each unique, and we must work to understand what makes them different.

The best clinicians are those who develop an appropriate, pragmatic, and individualized plan for managing concussion while effectively counseling the athlete, parent, and coach throughout the process. *Cram Session in Evaluation of Sports Concussion* can provide a head start in accomplishing these goals. It has the potential to become a classic guide for managing this ever so challenging injury—the sport-related concussion.

Kevin M. Guskiewicz, PhD, ATC
Kenan Distinguished Professor and Chair
Department of Exercise and Sport Science
Founding Director of the Matthew Gfeller Sport-
Related Traumatic Brain Injury Research Center
University of North Carolina—Chapel Hill
Chapel Hill, North Carolina

Introduction

This book was written with both former and new students in mind. Providing a minimalist approach with best evidence practices has been the most ideal way to teach this topic to undergraduates, graduate medical students, and clinicians. This philosophy has been continued in this book. I tried to develop and implement my teaching style, both didactically and clinically, and put it into book format. For my students (who *love* to read textbooks), I included organizational flow charts, concept maps, tables, and charts to provide a visual description of the process.

The difficulty in dealing with an entire book on concussion is the fluidity of concussion assessment and management techniques, research, and evidence. This book is not intended to be an all-encompassing answer to every clinical question that arises during the assessment and management of concussion. New assessment techniques are continuously being developed while new legislation and proposed treatment plans are being drafted. This book will hopefully be the first step of many to develop more standardized evaluation techniques and holistic management plans that include return to participation, school, and work following a concussive injury.

This book is primarily an evaluation book that focuses on how clinicians can develop differential diagnoses and then systematically rule each one in or out to come up with a final diagnosis. An entire chapter dedicated to all the differential diagnoses associated with concussion is included, signifying the importance of developing the differential diagnosis and confirming the diagnosis. Each differential diagnosis includes red flag boxes that necessitate immediate referral and key components to each diagnosis.

This book follows traditional chapter format that progresses from a brief introduction, discussion of differential diagnoses, step-by-step evaluation process, management and recovery, return to participation guidelines, school/work accomodations, legislation, and prevention. Each chapter then provides an overview, evidence to support each step in the process, and concluding summarized chapter bullets.

Tamerah N. Hunt, PhD, AT

INTRODUCTION

Historical Perspective

The media explosion involving sport-related concussions and the forced retirement of several high profile athletes such as Al Toon, Troy Aikman, Steve Young, and Eric Lindros provides helpful insight into the nature of concussion research, evaluation, and management. This chapter will begin by discussing the evolution of head injury description, evaluation, and awareness that has led to the modern day depiction of concussion.

Head injuries around the world have been described in various texts and documents throughout the ages. Modern concussion accounts revolve around the presentation of symptoms, cognitive dysfunction, and motor and behavioral changes (functional changes). Historically, typical descriptions of injuries described conditions such as seizures; paralysis; and loss of sight, hearing, or speech. A consistent diagnosis was not depicted.

Archeologists provided evidence of head injury management when they uncovered relics of skulls during digs in battle fields with holes drilled over fracture lines.[1] This practice of trephined skulls maintained throughout the ages as a way to alleviate humors (cerebral spinal fluid) and reduce pressure on the brain.[1] The first written document describing various head injuries and symptoms and classifying them on their presentation appears to be the Edwin Smith Papyrus (dated around 1650 to 1550 BC).[2]

Medical documents from Greece (specifically the Hippocratic Corpus), appears to be the first mention of *commotio cerebri*, or commotion of the brain, and is described symptomatically as a loss of speech, hearing, and sight.[3] This description of changes in mental function by "shaking of the brain" remained the leading theory accepted until the 19th century.[3]

In 900 AD a Persian physician, Abu Bakr Muhammad ibn Zakariya al-Razi, first discussed concussion as distinct from other types of head injury.[4] He appears to be the first physician to call the set of symptoms previously described as *cerebral concussion*. His definition was based upon the lack of physical damage with temporary loss of function. Additional support for concussion as a separate condition came from Guido Lanfrancus

Hunt TN.
*Cram Session in Evaluation of Sports Concussion:
A Handbook for Students & Clinicians* (pp. 1-17).
© 2013 Taylor & Francis Group.

in 1280 AD, who further described the shaking of the brain resulting in cerebral paralysis. These researchers' theories set the stage for the medical community's understanding of the condition.[5]

The widely accepted definition of Razi that the shaking of the brain, or *commotio*, led to clinical changes in the brain was widely accepted until the 17th century when the microscope was invented.[6,7] The microscope allowed physicians to examine the physical and structural mechanisms of injury. Microscopic evidence supported that the injury did not result from physical damage.[6,7] At this point, *concussion* was used to describe the state of unconsciousness and other functional problems.[6,7]

In the 18th century, understanding of concussion progressed when Thomas Kirkland documented that concussions were not structural injuries. This led to further clarification of the injury, which brought forth the modern description of a concussive injury.[8] The description and definition of concussion continued to become more specific over time, with a more thorough description of reported symptoms, understanding of the transient nature of the condition, the long-term sequelae of the injury, and presentation of *punch-drunk syndrome.*[9-12]

The 19th century saw the development of the first helmet (made primarily of leather), which was introduced to football in 1893. This invention demonstrated the importance of protecting the brain in sport.[13] The use of helmets became mandatory in football by the National Collegiate Athletic Association (NCAA) in 1939 and the National Football League (NFL) in 1940.[13]

The 20th century saw an upswing of media and head injury publicity. This century also noticed an increase in athletic participation, producing a greater numbers of exposures, which resulted in a greater risk for concussion. Traumatic brain injury (TBI) caused by trauma to the head grew to a public health concern in the 1970s. As a result, significant research involving brain trauma and pharmacological management of head injuries emerged in the 1990s. During this time, additional media publicity of concussions sustained by high profile athletes and military veterans returning from war encouraged technological support for traumatic brain injuries. The awareness and support for brain injuries resulted in the declaration of the 1990s as the *brain decade.*[14]

In the 21st century, the Centers for Disease Control (CDC) labeled concussion an epidemic and worked toward enhancing research and education, which led to the creation of the CDC Heads Up program in 2002.[14] The push for legislative support to prevent catastrophic brain injuries in sport resulted in the Zachery Lystedt law being signed in 2009. The NFL also initiated stricter concussion management guidelines in 2009. The support of the legislation, new rule enforcement, and the change in concussion management guidelines for concussed athletes from the NFL increased awareness and trickled down to other agencies such as the NCAA and the National Federation of State High School Associations (NFHS), among others.

Sport-related concussions have become a major concern in athletics at all levels. Direct and indirect medical costs from lost productivity as a result of TBI totaled an estimated $76.5 billion in the United States in 2000.[15] TBI is a contributing factor to one-third (30.5%) of all injury-related deaths in the United States.[16] With a heightened awareness conveyed through the media, many organizations have provided educational materials, position statements, and clinical care guidelines. However, much of this information has not been readily available to all practicing clinicians.

The seriousness of the condition has spurred major changes over the last several decades, including changes in equipment and changes to legislation regarding concussion management. Bridging the gap between research and clinical practice is the key to better management of sport-related concussion and improving return-to-play decisions.

Definition of Concussion

A book about concussion evaluation and management requires a discussion about the appropriate terminology and the inconsistency of the terminology that has been utilized. Concussions have been called mild TBI (MTBI), TBI, concussion, "ding," and/or "getting your bell rung." These terms are also typically used interchangeably. Unfortunately, using terms such as *getting your bell rung* and *ding* makes the perception of the injury much less serious. Studies have found that athletes' and coaches' perspective of the injury was dependent on the terminology utilized. Seventy percent of football players who were considered "dinged" returned to play in the same game or practice.[17,18] Additionally, coaches believed that loss of consciousness must occur to diagnose a concussion when less than 10% of concussive injuries actually include a loss of consciousness.[17] The confusion of the injury nomenclature reduces the significance of the injury. This has led to experts involved in the Third International Conference on Concussion in Sport in 2008 to suggest that clinicians maintain a separation from MTBI and concussion as 2 entities because the terms refer to different injury constructs and should not be used interchangeably. From this point forward, this book will use the term *concussion* to refer to sport-related concussive injuries.[19]

In addition to the ambiguity over what to call the injury, it was only recently that a consensus agreement had been adapted regarding the definition of concussion. Previous definitions were based on loss of consciousness and amnesia and, at times, were synonymous with a contusion to the brain.[20] Literature has provided conclusive evidence that these 2 commonly utilized markers were not required for the injury to be considered a concussion.[21-23]

The traditional approach to severe TBI had been to utilize on-field loss of consciousness (LOC) as the primary measure of injury severity. Findings in this field describe LOC in association with specific early deficits, but LOC does not necessarily imply severity.[19,21] As such, the presence of LOC as a symptom would not necessarily classify the concussion as complex or indicate the severity of concussive injuries.[19,22] However, it is difficult to "get the word out" about what a concussion is and is not when the definition and key elements are continually changing.

Concussions in athletic populations appear to result in transient symptoms of short duration. Concussion comes from the Latin term *concutere*, meaning "to strike together." Concussion was originally defined in 1966 by the committee of Head Injury Nomenclature of the Congress of Neurological Surgeons as "a graded set of clinical symptoms that may or may not involve LOC. Resolution of the clinical and cognitive symptoms typically follows a sequential course."[23,24]

Prior to the Head Injury Nomenclature of the Congress of Neurological Surgeons' definition, the 2 most popular cited definitions were based on functional status and the nature of medical signs and symptoms present at the time of injury.[25] However, these definitions were found to be vague and ambiguous, causing confusion for physicians and allied medical practitioners associated with concussion assessment.[23] Experts, clinicians, and researchers in the field have recently come to a consensus regarding the definition of concussion as "a complex pathophysiological process affecting the brain, induced by traumatic biomechanical forces."[25(p6)] The consensus from the first International Conference on Concussion in Sport in 2001 suggested the following 5 conditions of concussion[23,25]:

1. Concussion may be caused either by a direct blow to the head, face, neck, or elsewhere on the body with an "impulsive" or rotational force transmitted to the head.
2. Concussion typically results in the rapid onset of short-lived impairment of neurological function that resolves spontaneously.
3. Concussion may result in neuropathological changes, but the acute clinical symptoms rarely reflect a functional disturbance rather than structural injury.

4. Concussion results in a graded set of clinical syndromes that may or may not involve LOC; resolution of the clinical and cognitive symptoms typically follows a sequential course.
5. Concussion is typically associated with normal structural neuroimaging studies.[23]

Epidemiology

The number of concussions has reached overwhelming rates in contact sports at both the professional and amateur levels. Within sports at all levels, it appears that 5% to 40% of all injuries are concussions.[26-30] Previously 300,000 concussions annually were cited[27-29]; however, it was later found that this figure was the number of concussions seen only in emergency departments. Currently, there are an estimated 1.6 to 3.8 million sport-related concussions occurring in the United States annually.[31]

The CDC recently proclaimed that concussions in athletes have reached an epidemic level in the United States.[14] Although the incidence of life-threatening brain injury has decreased in most sports, there is more recent evidence suggesting that concussion may be more common and more serious than previously thought.[23,29,32-34] Between 1982 and 2002, brain injury was a primary cause of 551 deaths among roughly 120 million high school and college athletes.[32] The numbers attributed to concussion have recently been questioned, as incidents of concussion may be under-reported.[33]

Several factors (ie, age, gender, and player position) are associated with the incidence and reporting of concussive injuries. While research and clinical care is usually focused on contact sports like football, rugby, and ice hockey, concussive injuries occur in all sports. The rates vary based on several aspects though the most common are type of sport, gender of players, and type of exposure. If the clinician is aware of injury rates, patterns of injury, and associated risk factors, he or she can provide preventative care and targeted interventions to reduce the risk of concussions in all athletes, thereby making participation safe for everyone involved.

Age

Children between the ages of 6 and 16 years are 6 times more likely to sustain a concussion while playing organized sports than during recreational activities.[24,25] In a traditional competitive football season, Guskiewicz et al[28] found that 5% of all collegiate athletes receive a concussion, while there is variable evidence that reports approximately 5% to 20% of high school athletes receive a concussion. McCrea et al[33] found a prevalence of 15.3% in high school athletics. This rate is 3 times the amount of collegiate athletes. Additionally, 80% of youth concussions are considered mild concussions and more than half go unreported to medical personnel.[22]

In rugby, concussive injuries accounted for 25% of injuries resulting in loss of playing or training time in the under-13-years age group.[34-36] Powell and Barber-Foss[37] conducted a study that examined 246 high schools and found that almost 90% of high school athletes surveyed had sustained at least one concussion during their athletic career. Approximately 10% sustained 2 concussions and fewer than 1% sustained 3 or more concussions during their career. The study also found that high school athletes with 3 or more concussions are 9 times more likely to have more severe on-field presentation in subsequent injuries.[37]

Gender

Evidence suggests that gender may also play a role in concussion incidence.[38-42] Female athletes appear to have a higher incidence of concussion compared to their male counterparts. Borowski et al[38] found a concussion rate among female high school soccer players to be 68% higher than among males. This study also compared high school basketball players and found that female athletes report triple the rate of concussion injuries compared to male athletes. According to the NCAA surveillance data, women's ice hockey had the highest incidence of concussions (18.1%) in collegiate sports, followed by men's ice hockey (7.9%), women's lacrosse (6.3%), and football (6.0%).[29]

While incidence and rate of concussion depend heavily on self-reporting, there is evidence that females are more honest in reporting general injuries than males.[40,41] Further, poor neck strength has been associated with gender differences.[42] It is unclear whether the concussion incidence data—while generally consistent in showing a higher risk in females as compared to males in similar sports—is a true difference or is influenced by a reporting bias.[40] The lack of objective tools, consistent symptoms and definitions, and biological markers to indicate concussive injuries can bias accurate injury data.

Player Position

Research suggests that many concussive injuries happen while tackling or being tackled.[43] Powell and Barber-Foss[37] found that high school football linebackers, running backs, and offensive lineman had the most incidences of concussion. In rugby, it appears that midfield back, inside back, and back row player positions had the highest rate of concussion in professional rugby, while soccer players found greater concussion incidence in midfielders.[42]

Overall, these positions appear to be involved with tackling. The ability to educate and coach proper tackling technique may indeed be advantageous in the prevention of concussion.

While incidence rates are variable, they do appear to be affected by age, gender, bias in reporting, willingness to report injuries, and location of contact or injury. Clinicians working with athletes should encourage honest and accurate reporting of symptoms to ensure a proper evaluation is conducted to prevent worse outcomes following injury.

Basic Anatomy

It is important to recognize and understand the structural support and basic anatomy of the brain and how it relates to a concussive injury. Figure 1-1 shows basic brain anatomy. The first line of support is represented by the bony anatomy of the skull.

The Skull

The skull is designed for maximal protection of the brain. This protection is obtained by the combination of multiple flat bones (frontal, occipital, temporal, and parietal) that form together at sutures, that harden as a function of age. The bones of the skull are very dense. The density decreases that amount of physical shock transmitted to the brain. Lastly, the skull provides an attachment site for the skin, providing an additional layer of protection to cushion and disseminate forces transmitted to the brain.[44]

The structure of the brain and mechanism of injury provide a glimpse into the variability of the injury. This section provides a quick review of the basic brain anatomy and functions as they relate to concussive injuries. The major regions of the brain consist of the brainstem, diencephalon, the cerebrum (which is divided into 2 hemispheres), and the cerebellum. Each region is responsible for vital cognitive, motor, sensory, and balance functions. While there is some overlap in function, each region is responsible for a set of functions and will be described in more detail in the following paragraphs.

Brainstem

The brainstem consists of the medulla oblongata, pons, and midbrain.[44,45] The brainstem connects the spinal cord to the brain and is typically associated with responsibility of essential survival functions (see Figure 1-1). The medulla oblongata is the most inferior portion of the brainstem and regulates heart rate, blood vessel diameter, breathing, swallowing, vomiting, coughing, and sneezing. The pons is located immediately superior to the

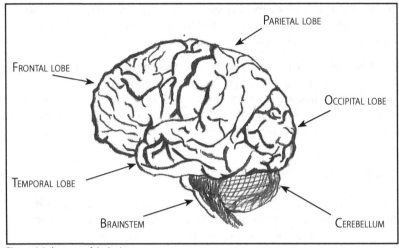

Figure 1-1. Anatomy of the brain.

medulla oblongata and relays information between the cerebrum and the cerebellum by means of nuclei and nerve tracts. The midbrain is superior to the pons and plays a role in hearing and vision. Collectively, the brainstem also houses the reticular activating system, which is involved in arousing and maintaining consciousness.

Diencephalon

The diencephalon houses the thalamus and hypothalamus.[44,45] Ascending sensory nerve tracts synapse in the thalamus. It is also responsible for influencing mood and registering discomfort, or the perception of pain. The hypothalamus is responsible for maintaining homeostasis. Most common features associated with the hypothalamus are the control of body temperature, hunger, and thirst.

Cerebrum

The cerebrum is the largest portion of the brain and is divided into lobes named for the bones that lie above them.[44,45] The frontal lobe is vital for voluntary motor function, motivation, aggression, and mood. It is commonly associated with executive functions that include information processing, attention, memory, inhibition, and impulse control. The parietal lobe is the principal center for reception and evaluation of pain, temperature, pressure (touch), and taste. The occipital lobe controls functions of reception and integration of visual input, and the temporal lobe is responsible for smell, auditory input, and memory.

Cerebellum

The cerebellum is the most posterior portion of the brain and is easily identifiable by the visible striations and presence of grey matter.[44,45] The cerebellum is responsible for balance, maintenance of muscle tone, and coordination of fine motor movement.

Therefore, depending on the location of injury in the brain, those with a concussive injury can sustain observed motor, sensory, cognitive, and behavioral deficits.

Mechanism of Injury

Coup/Contrecoup Model

There are several noted mechanisms for concussion. The most common mechanism in sport-related concussion is the coup/contrecoup model.[21,46,47] In the coup/contrecoup model, the skull moves in a direction until it is stopped by the physical limitations of the neck tissues. When this happens, the brain continues to move until it is acted upon by an outside force (the skull). While the cerebral spinal fluid will offer some resistance to motion, it is often not enough. As such, the brain will make contact with the interior of the skull, causing a concussion.[23]

The initial site of contact is called a *coup injury*. This can result in mechanical damage to the brain at the point of contact.[23] Coup injuries occur when the site of damage is associated with a direct blow. This typically results in a contusion or focal lesions that affect specific functions of the brain in relation to the injured area.

If the brain were to then rebound into the opposite side of the skull, a contrecoup injury would result. Structural deformation can result at both points of contact. This type of injury commonly results from a direct impact to the head, either to the frontal or occipital bones.[23] In contrecoup injuries, the injured site is where the brain bounces around inside the skull, resulting in multiple areas of injury. These focal lesions tend to cross over multiple functions and can be predicted by the location of impact.

Rotational Forces

Another mechanism that could lead to more severe injuries is caused by a rotational component. A diffuse axonal injury will result from uncontrolled head rotation. In this model, the lateral rotation of the head causes stretching of the cerebral neurons. Ommaya et al[48] proposed the centripetal theory of injury, which states that the most superficial neurons sustain the greatest level of insult, and the degree of injury decreases toward the rotational center of the brain. The result of a diffuse axonal injury is a stretching of the neurons; the brain does not come in contact with the internal cranium.[48] The stretching, if severe enough, has the potential to tear some tissues and vessels, but is more likely to result in a depolarization of the neurons.[23]

Repeated Subconcussive Forces

Many athletic pursuits provide an opportunity for contact and trauma. Numerous hits may occur and clinicians are unaware of whether the force from the hit can cause a concussion. Researchers are beginning to examine the possibility of quantifying the force it takes to sustain a concussion.[49,50] New technological advances, such as accelerometers in helmets, provide the means to understand the amount of force it takes to produce a concussion through contact in sports. Commonly reported[49,50] forces occurring during contact in football studies have been reported to be 80 to 90 gravitational forces (g). However, impact forces greater than 90 g without the presence of symptoms did not result in concussion.[49] Further, only 35% of impacts greater than 80 g resulted in concussion.[49,50] During identification of concussion in biomechanical research, impact forces are classified as *above* concussion threshold and *below* concussion threshold.

Several studies have been published examining the gravitational forces associated with collegiate American football.[49-54] Duma et al[51] found a mean peak linear acceleration of the head of 32 g. Many studies examine the concussion threshold, or more specifically, determine the acceleration forces of the head when concussions occur as the clinical outcome.[51-54] As early as 1982, Hugenholtz and Richard[52] proposed that concussion resulted from a blow to the head equivalent to a linear acceleration 80 to 90 times the force of gravity for more than 4 ms. Pellman et al[53] published a series of studies based on concussive injuries occurring during professional football games. This group used video data to reconstruct the angle, speed, and resultant player kinematics of the injury to propose a potential injury threshold of 70 to 75 g. Additional studies have observed concussive injury with peak linear accelerations ranging from the low 60s to 80 g. Although Pellman et al[53] suggested a 75% injury tolerance level for impacts above 98 g, Guskiewicz et al[55] found only a 0.3% injury tolerance for impacts above 80 g.

It appears that within the research,[49-56] forces greater than 60 g can be implicated for concussive injuries. In collegiate athletes 1% of hits were above the concussion threshold, while 0.7% of hits were above the concussion threshold in high school athletes.[54] As 99% of hits obtained were below concussion threshold, very little is known about the physiological effects of subthreshold forces or normal repetitive contact on cognition.[54]

Until recently there were conflicting data as to whether repetitive sub-concussive forces associated with purposely heading the ball in soccer are a cause of long-term health problems.[56] Putukian et al[57] followed college soccer players for one season to perform neuropsychological testing. The number of heading contacts and minutes played were also counted for all home games by team athletic trainers and physicians. It was found that male, college-aged players had an average of 0.783 headers/minute during a single season and females had an average of 0.753 headers/minute.[58] Many studies[56-60] provide evidence that purposeful heading does not increase the incidence of concussion in soccer players. Understanding the biomechanics of these forces provides useful information regarding when to remove a player from sport, what type of forces can be prevented with protective equipment, and which levels of forces are traumatic.

Physiologic Mechanism (Metabolic Cascade)

Physiologic mechanism research began in animal models, particularly rats.[61-63] Following a concussive blow, massive depolarization of cells create a release of glutamine requiring increased adenosine triphosphate (ATP) and glucose.[61-63] Because of the increased use of ATP to maintain the now-disturbed potassium balance and membrane potential, glucose utilization is increased through glycolysis, which creates a state of hyperglycolysis. This may last up to 30 minutes in rats. The cerebral blood flow may not meet demand with uncoupling of brain cells.[62,63] This glucose metabolism depression may last 7 to 10 days.[64,65]

After humans sustain a blow to the head, the neurons of the brain are stretched to the point where mechanical deformation takes place and the voltage-gated channels within the membrane are opened.[66] The brain experiences a sudden neuronal depolarization that leads to an indiscriminate triggering of voltage-dependent channels, thereby releasing several excitatory amino acids, the main one being glutamate. Glutamate begins a neurometabolic cascade that leads to ionic shifts and chemical changes within the brain.[67] Glutamate binds with N-Nitrosodimethylamine receptors that, in turn, open channels by which potassium (K^+) and calcium (Ca^{2+}) efflux and influx, respectively.[23,67] Magnetic resonance (MR) spectroscopy demonstrate a metabolic change with decrease in N-acetylaspartate and a significant decrease in glutamate following concussion.[68]

In response to injury, brain blood flow decreases by up to 50%.[69] The increase in extracellular K^+ triggers membrane sodium-potassium pumps to attempt restoration of homeostasis.[69] Increased pump action requires ATP, so glycolysis is sent into overdrive in an attempt to meet the energy demand.[67] This takes place in an oxygen-starved environment because cerebral blood flow has been reduced.[23]

The increase in extracellular K^+ has a negative effect on mitochondrial ability to perform normal oxidative capacities.[67] This, in turn, further elevates the energy crisis within the brain. Once extracellular K^+ has begun to decrease, the brain begins to experience further metabolic slowing. This slowing has been termed *spreading depression*.[67] The condition has been affiliated with decreases in neuronal firing, which leads to neurocognitive dysfunction.[23]

Giza and Hovda[68] reported that extracellular K^+ increases quickly after the onset of injury but decreases back to normal levels within 30 minutes. Elevated levels of K^+ have been related to decreased mitochondrial function and propagation of the energy deficit by triggering sodium-potassium pump response.[68] Ca^{2+}, on the other hand, remains at elevated levels from 2 to 4 days post-injury. Elevated levels of Ca^{2+} have been attributed to neuronal disconnection and cell death.[23]

A by-product of the energy crises is the over-production and build-up of lactate. Too much lactate can cause a change in the pH of the surrounding area, which has been shown to damage cellular membranes, thereby increasing brain vulnerability.[67] Over time this process will correct itself.[23]

It appears that adults return to normal following a sport-related concussion in about 3 days.[70] Decreased cerebral brain flow, as documented in humans, has been shown to last up to 10 days. Unfortunately, recent research involving positron emission topography (PET) scans provide evidence of increased glucose demand followed by glucose depression and metabolic recovery that may last for weeks to months.[71] The condition decreases brain metabolism, which has been related to neuronal dysfunction and decreases in brain function (ie, neurocognitive function and possibly motor control). The condition is also thought to place the brain into a state of vulnerability where it cannot respond to injury or hyperactivity, therefore increasing the risk for a second concussive injury. This increased risk is supported by research that found concussed athletes are up to 6 times more likely to get a second concussion than nonconcussed athletes.[23,72]

Summary

- Head injuries can be traced back through the centuries with specific references to concussions in the 10th century.

- The clinical characteristics of concussion have been described similarly. Until recently, ambiguity regarding the terminology of concussion decreased the importance and potential outcomes associated with this condition.

- The injury does not result in structural changes but rather in functional deficits based on the location and mechanism of the injury.

- The anatomy of the brain plays an important role in understanding the underlying physiological and behavioral changes as a result of the structures that are injured.

- Concussion is a hypermetabolic disorder that results when the energy available does not meet the brain's energy needs.

- Concussive injuries occur in all sports, regardless of age and gender. Higher incidences are reported in contact sports (eg, ice hockey, football, soccer, and lacrosse), younger athletes, and female athletes.

- Understanding the historical, anatomical, and physiological side of concussive injuries provides support for evaluation and management of concussive injuries.

References

1. Scurlock JA, Andersen BR. *Diagnoses in Assyrian and Babylonian Medicine: Ancient Sources, Translations, and Modern Medical Analyses.* Urbana, IL: University of Illinois Press; 2005:307.

2. Sanchez GM, Burridge AL. Decision making in head injury management in the Edwin Smith Papyrus. *Neurosurg Focus.* 2007;23(1):1-9.

3. Levin HS, Benton AL, Grossman R. Historical review of head injury. In: *Neurobehavioral Consequences of Closed Head Injury.* Oxford, Oxfordshire: Oxford University Press; 1982:3-5.

4. Souayah N, Greenstein JI. Insights into neurologic localization by Rhazes, a medieval Islamic physician. *Neurology.* 2005;65(1):125-128.

5. McHenry L. *Garrison's History of Neurology.* Springfield, IL: Charles C Thomas; 1969:1-23.

6. Zillmer EA, Schneider J, Tinker J, Kaminaris CI. A history of sports-related concussions: a neuropsychological perspective. In: Echemendia RJ, ed. *Sports Neuropsychology: Assessment and Management of Traumatic Brain Injury.* New York, NY: The Guilford Press; 2006:21-23.

7.   Corcoran C, McAlister TW, Malaspina D. Psychotic disorders. In: Silver JM, McAllister TW, Yudofsky SC, eds. *Textbook of Traumatic Brain Injury*. Washington, DC: American Psychiatric Association; 2005:189-199.

8.   Kirkland T. *A Commentary on Apoplectic and Paralytic Affections and on Diseases Connected With the Subject*. London: William Dawson; 1792.

9.   Abernathy J. *On Injuries of the Head. Surgical and Physiological Works*. Vol 2. London: Longman, Ress, Orme, Brown and Green; 1830.

10. Erichsen J. *The Science and Art of Surgery*. 10th ed. London: Longmans Green; 1895;23-31.

11. Martland H. Punch drunk. *J Amer Med Assoc*. 1928;91:1103-1107.

12. Romanis W, Mitchiner P. *The Science and Practice of Surgery*. Vol 2. 5th ed. Philadelphia, PA: Lea and Febiger; 1934:1-45.

13. Levy M, Ozgur B, Berry C, Aryan HE, Apuzzo ML. Birth and evolution of the football helmet. *Neurosurgery*. 2004;55:656-662.

14. Centers for Disease Control and Prevention. Sports-related recurrent brain injuries, United States. *MMWR Morb Mortal Wkly Rep*. 1997;46:224-227.

15. Finkelstein EA, Corso PS, Miller TR. *The Incidence and Economic Burden of Injuries in the United States*. New York, NY: Oxford University Press; 2006.

16. Centers for Disease Control and Prevention. *Report to Congress on Mild Traumatic Brain Injury in the United States: Steps to Prevent a Serious Public Health Problem*. Atlanta (GA): Centers for Disease Control and Prevention, National Center for Injury Prevention and Control; 2003.

17. Valovich McLeod TC, Bay RC, Heil J, McVeigh SD. Identification of sport and recreational activity concussion history through the pre-participation screening and a symptom survey in young athletes. *Clin J Sport Med*. 2008;18:235-240.

18. Shulz MR, Marshall SW, Mueller FO, et al. Incidence and risk factors for concussion in high school athletes, North Carolina, 1996–1999. *Am J Epidemiol*. 2004;160(10):937-944.

19. McCrory P, Meeuwisse W, Johnston K, et al. Consensus statement on concussion in sport, 3rd international conference on concussion in sport. Zurich 2008. *Clin J Sport Med*. 2009;19:185-200.

20. Kelly JP, Nichols JS, Filley CM, Lillehei CO, Rubinstein D, Kleinschmidt-DeMasters BK. Concussion in sports: guidelines for the prevention of catastrophic outcome. *JAMA*. 1991;266(20):2867-2869.

21. Bailes JE, Cantu RC. Head injury in athletes. *Neurosurgery*. 2001;48(1):26-42.

22. Sherer M, Struchen MA, Yablon SA, Wang Y, Nick TG. Comparison of indices of traumatic brain injury severity: Glasgow Coma Scale, length of coma and post-traumatic amnesia. *J Neurol Neurosurg Psychiatry*. 2008;79(6):678-685.

23. Hunt TN. The psychometric properties of concussion assessment tools in high school athletics [dissertation]. Athens, GA: University of Georgia; 2006.

24. Esselman PC, Uomoto JM. Classification of the spectrum of mild traumatic brain injury. *Brain Injury*. 1995;9:417-424.

25. Aubry M, Cantu R, Dvorak J, et al. Summary and agreement statement of the First International Conference on Concussion in Sport, Vienna 2001: recommendations for the improvement of safety and health of athletes who may suffer concussive injuries. *Br J Sports Med*. 2002;36(1):6-10.

26. Hootman JM, Dick R, Agel J. Epidemiology of collegiate injuries in 15 sports: summary and recommendations for injury prevention initiatives. *J Athl Train*. 2007;42(2):311-319.

27. Gerberich SG, Priest JD, Boen JR, Straub CP, Maxwell RE. Concussion incidences and severity in secondary school varsity football players. *Am J Public Health.* 1983;73(12):1370-1375.

28. Guskiewicz KM, Weaver NL, Padua DA, et al. Epidemiology of concussion in collegiate and high school football players. *Am J Sports Med.* 2000;28(5):643-650.

29. Marar M, McIlvain NM, Fields SK, Comstock RD. Epidemiology of concussions among United States high school athletes in 20 sports. *Am J Sports Med.* 2012;40:1231-1233.

30. Cantu RC. Head and spine injuries in the young athlete. *Clin Sports Med.* 1988;7(3):459-472.

31. Thurman D, Branche C, Sniezek JE. The epidemiology of sports-related traumatic brain injuries in the United States: recent developments. *J Head Trauma Rehabil.* 1998;13:1-8.

32. Langlois JA, Rutland-Brown W, Wald M. The epidemiology and impact of traumatic brain injury: a brief overview. *J Head Trauma Rehabil.* 2006;21(5):375-378.

33. McCrea M, Hammeke T, Olsen G, Leo P, Guskiewicz K. Unreported concussion in high school football players: implications for prevention. *Clin J Sport Med.* 2004;14(1):13-17.

34. Cassidy JD, Carroll LD, Peloso PM, et al. Incidence, risk factors and prevention of mild traumatic brain injury: results of the WHO collaborating centre task force on mild traumatic brain injury. *J Rehabil Med.* 2004;43(suppl):28-60.

35. Browne G, Lam L. Concussive head injury in children and adolescents related to sports and other leisure physical activities. *Br J Sports Med.* 2006;40:163-168.

36. McIntosh AS, McCrory P. Preventing head and neck injury. *Br J Sports Med.* 2005;39(6):314-318.

37. Powell JW, Barber-Foss KD. Traumatic brain injury in high school athletes. *JAMA.* 1999;282(10):958-963.

38. Borowski LA, Yard EE, Fields SK, Comstock RD. The epidemiology of US high school basketball injuries, 2005-2007. *Am J Sports Med.* 2008;36:2328-2335.

39. Dick RW. Is there a gender difference in concussion incidence and outcomes? *Br J Sports Med.* 2009;43(suppl 1):46-50.

40. Frommer LJ, Gurka KK, Cross KM, Ingersoll CD, Comstock RD, Saliba SA. Sex differences in concussion symptoms of high school athletes. *J Athl Train.* 2011;46(1):76-84.

41. Tierney RT, Sitler MR, Swanik CB, Swanik KA, Higgins M, Torg J. Gender differences in head-neck segment dynamic stabilization during head acceleration. *Med Sci Sports Exer.* 2005;37(2):272-279.

42. Gessel LM, Fields SK, Collins CL, Dick RW, Comstock RD. Concussions among United States high school and collegiate athletes. *J Athl Train.* 2007;42(4):495-503.

43. McIntosh AS, McCrory P, Finch CF, Wolfe R. Head, face and neck injury in youth rugby: incidence and risk factors. *Br J Sports Med.* 2010;44(3):188-193.

44. Moore KL. *Clinically Oriented Anatomy.* 3rd ed. Baltimore, MD: Williams & Wilkins; 1992:637-783.

45. McMinn R, Gaddum-Rosse P, Hutchings RT, Logan BM. *McMinn's Functional and Clinical Anatomy.* Barcelona: Mosby; 1995:193-213.

46. Cantu RC. Cerebral concussion in sport. *Sports Med.* 1992;17:64-74.

47. Cantu RC. Athletic head injuries. *Clin Sports Med.* 1997;17(1):37-43.

48. Ommaya AK, Goldsmith W, Thibault L. Biomechanics and neuropathology of adult and pediatric head injury. *Br J Neurosurgery.* 2002;16(3):220-242.

49. McCaffrey MA, Mihalik JP, Crowell DH, Shields EW, Guskiewicz KM. Measurement of head impacts in collegiate football players: clinical measurements of concussion after high- and low-magnitude impacts. *Neurosurgery.* 2007;61(6):1236-1243.

50. Mihalik JP, Bell DR, Marshall SW, Guskiewicz KM. Measurement of head impacts in collegiate football players: an investigation of positional and event-type difference. *Neurosurgery.* 2007;61(6):1229-1235.

51. Duma SM, Manoogian SJ, Bussone WR, et al. Analysis of real-time head accelerations in collegiate football players. *Clin Sports Med.* 2005;15:3-8.

52. Hugenholtz H, Richard MT. Return to athletic competition following concussion. *Can Med Assoc J.* 1982;127:827-829.

53. Pellman EJ, Viano DC, Tucker AM, Casson IR, Waeckerle JF. Concussion in professional football: reconstruction of game impacts and injuries. *Neurosurgery.* 2003;53:799-814.

54. Schnebel B, Gwin JT, Anderson S, Gatlin R. In vivo study of head impacts in football: a comparison of National Collegiate Athletic Association Division I versus high school impacts. *Neurosurgery.* 2006;60(3):490-496.

55. Guskiewicz KM, Mihalik JP, Shankar V, et al. Measurement of head impacts in collegiate football players: relationship between head impact biomechanics and acute clinical outcome after concussion. *Neurosurgery.* 2007;61:1244-1252.

56. Tysvaer AT, Lochen EA. Soccer injuries to the brain: a neuropsychologic study of former soccer players. *Am J Sports Med.* 1991;19(1):56-60.

57. Putukian M. Heading in soccer: is it safe? *Curr Sports Med Rep.* 2004;3(1):9-14.

58. Barnes BC, Cooper L, Kirkendall DT, et al. Concussion history in elite male and female soccer players. *Am J Sports Med.* 1998;26(3):433-438.

59. Guskiewicz KM, Marshall SW, Broglio SP, Cantu RC, Kirkendall DT. No evidence of impaired neurocognitive performance in collegiate soccer players. *Am J Sports Med.* 2002;30(2):157-162.

60. Kirkendall DT, Jordan SE, Garrett WE. Heading and head injuries in soccer. *Sports Med.* 2001;31(5):369-386.

61. Katayama Y, Becker DP, Tamura T, Hovda DA. Massive increases in extracellular potassium and the indiscriminate release of glutamate following concussive brain injury. *Neurosurgery.* 1990;73:889-900.

62. Kawamata T, Katayama Y, Hovda DA, Yoshino A, Becker DP. Administration of excitatory amino acid antagonists via microdialysis attenuates the increase in glucose utilization seen following concussive brain injury. *J Cereb Blood Flow Metab.* 1992;12:12-24.

63. Yoshino A, Hovda DA, Kawamata T, Katayama Y, Becker DP. Dynamic changes in local cerebral glucose utilization following cerebral conclusion in rats: evidence of a hyper- and subsequent hypometabolic state. *Brain Res.* 1991;561:106-119.

64. Kelly DF, Kozlowsji DA, Haddad E, Echiverri A, Hovda DA, Lee SM. Ethanol reduces metabolic uncoupling following experimental head injury. *J Neurotrauma.* 2000;17(5):261-272.

65. Kelly DF, Martin NA, Kordestani R, et al. Cerebral blood flow as a predictor of outcome following traumatic brain injury. *J Neurosurg.* 1997;86:241-251.

66. Hovda DA. Metabolic dysfunction. In: *Neurotrauma.* New York, NY: McGraw-Hill; 1996;1459-1478.

67. Giza CC, Hovda DA. The neurometabolic cascade of concussion. *J Athl Train.* 2001;36(3):228-235.

68. Henry LC, Trembley S, Boulanger Y, Ellemberg D, Lassonde M. Neurometabolic changes in the acute phase after sports concussion correlate with symptom severity. *J Neurotrauma.* 2010;27(1):65-76.

69. Hovda DA, Villablanca JR. Cerebral metabolism following neonatal or adult hemineo-decortication in cats: effect on oxidative capacity using cytochrome oxidase histochemistry. *Brain Res Dev Brain Res.* 1998;110(1):39-50.

70. Guskiewicz KM, Ross SE, Marshall SW. Postural stability and neuropsychological deficits after concussion in collegiate athletes. *J Athl Train.* 2001;36(3):263-273.

71. Bergsneider M, Hovda DA, Lee SM, et al. Dissociation of cerebral glucose metabolism and level of consciousness during the period of metabolic depression following human traumatic brain injury. *J Neurotrauma.* 2000;17(5):389-401.

72. Cantu RC. Posttraumatic retrograde and anterograde amnesia: pathophysiology and implications in grading and safe return to play. *J Athl Train.* 2001;36(3):244-248.

DIFFERENTIAL DIAGNOSES

During an evaluation, clinicians spend the majority of their time determining the diagnosis of the injury. In the process of evaluation, clinicians consider other diagnoses that could possibly result in the same signs and symptoms. These are commonly called *differential diagnoses*. The clinician then focuses the remaining portion of the evaluation on ruling in or out each differential diagnosis during the evaluation process.

The most common diagnoses associated with head injuries are epidural hematoma, subdural hematoma, skull fracture, second impact syndrome, post-concussion syndrome, seizure disorder, stroke, and exertional heat illness. From 1945 to 1999, there were 712 fatalities resulting from football injuries, with head injuries accounting for 69% of that total.[1] These fatalities have been attributed to epidural and subdural hematoma, second impact syndrome (SIS), and skull fractures.

This chapter will focus on how to differentiate between these conditions and concussion. The definition and common signs and symptoms of injury at presentation and differential guides will be presented for each condition.

Hunt TN.
*Cram Session in Evaluation of Sports Concussion:
A Handbook for Students & Clinicians* (pp. 19-34).
© 2013 Taylor & Francis Group.

Hematomas

Hematomas are localized collections of blood and spinal fluid in the space underneath the outer covering of the brain (dura), usually resulting from a laceration in the brain and/or tear in a blood vessel.[2] Hematomas are commonly divided into 2 major types in athletics: subdural and epidural.[3] Hematomas are considered a medical emergency and should be immediately referred to the emergency department once suspected.

Epidural Hematoma

An epidural hematoma is arterial bleeding between the inner bones of the skull and the dura mater.[3] Epidural hematomas often result from a tear of the artery, most often in the middle meningeal artery. Epidural hematomas present with rapid deterioration in functions, especially cognitive and behavioral. In sports, these injuries are typically associated with the degree of impact that results in a skull fracture.

- **Onset:** The onset of symptoms for an epidural hematoma is rapid. The symptoms occur within minutes to hours of the injury. The athlete may come off the playing surface and report severe or incredible pain.

RED FLAG FOR DIAGNOSIS
Epidural Hematoma

- ⦿ Cognitive deterioration within minutes to hours
- ⦿ Increasing headache

- **Pain:** Pain is traditionally reported as headache or is caused by resultant bruising based on the mechanism of injury. The most telling sign of epidural hematoma is a headache that worsens over time.

- **Mechanism of injury:** Trauma that results from a blow to the head or body that jars the brain or a coup/contrecoup mechanism.

- **Observation:** Patient may have loss of consciousness that progresses to a period of lucidity and then rapidly deteriorates to a loss of consciousness as the hematoma forms. Look for bruising or ecchymosis behind the mastoid process (battle signs) and around the eyes (raccoon eyes), which are indicative of a skull fracture. Pupils may dilate on affected side.

- **Palpation:** Generally no areas are tender to palpation unless there is a secondary contusion resulting from the mechanism of injury. Palpation should include skull, sinus, orbital bone, and relevant musculature (eg, sternocleidomastoid, scalene, and trapezius musculature).

- **Range of motion:** Active, passive, and resistive range of motion will be within normal limits. Lateral rotation of the head may cause vertigo.

- **Signs and symptoms:** Disorientation, confusion, decline in cognitive function, abnormal behavior (eg, overly aggressive, combative, or emotional), complaints of drowsiness, and increasing headache.

- **Neurological testing:** Upper quarter screen and cranial nerve testing should be performed. Cranial nerve testing is normal unless hematoma formation presses directly against the brain and cranial nerves.

- **Special tests:** Vertebral artery test and Romberg test should be conducted.

- **Diagnosis:** Final diagnosis is typically confirmed with computed tomography (CT). If you suspect an epidural hematoma, this is a medical emergency. Refer immediately to the emergency department.

Subdural Hematoma

A subdural hematoma usually results from a tear in the veins that connect the surface of the cortex to the dura mater.[2] Subdural hematomas are further divided into the following 2 categories:

1. Simple—Not associated with direct cerebral damage.
2. Complex—Associated with contusions of the brain's surface and associated swelling.

- **Onset:** The onset of symptoms for a subdural hematoma is slower than an epidural hematoma. Symptoms typically present over hours, days, or weeks after the injury.

RED FLAG FOR DIAGNOSIS
Subdural Hematoma

- ◉ Deterioration of cognition
- ◉ Deterioration of posture and behavior over time
- ◉ Symptoms do not improve

- **Pain:** Pain is traditionally reported as headache or is caused by resultant bruising based on the mechanism of injury. The most telling signs of subdural hematoma are headache or behavioral changes (ie, uncharacteristic emotions) that worsen as the hematoma increases in size, pressing against vital structures. This may occur over several days.

- **Mechanism of injury:** Trauma that results from a blow to the head or body that jars the brain or a coup/contrecoup mechanism.

- **Observation:** There is a period of improvement, then a period of deterioration over days to weeks. The delayed onset of symptoms results in the clinical presentation of an athlete who does not recall the incident that could have caused the hematoma. Look for bruising or ecchymosis behind the mastoid process (battle signs) and around the eyes (raccoon eyes), which are indicative of a skull fracture. Pupils may dilate on affected side. Observe skin color and temperature, as well, if the athlete is in obvious pain.

- **Palpation:** Generally, no areas are tender to palpation unless there is a contusion resulting from the mechanism of injury. Palpation should include skull, sinus, orbital region, and musculature (eg, sternocleidomastoid, scalene, and trapezius musculature).

- **Range of motion:** Active, passive, and resistive range of motion will be within normal limits and of normal quality.

- **Signs and symptoms:** Drowsiness, confusion, headache, apathy, and a decreasing level of consciousness.

- **Neurological testing:** The athlete will present with normal intact upper and lower quarter screen initially following injury. As hematoma formation continues, there will be a marked decrease in the patient's motor, sensation, and reflex testing. Cranial nerve assessment is normal unless hematoma formation presses directly against the brain and cranial nerve.

- **Special tests:** Vertebral artery test and Romberg test should be conducted.

- **Diagnosis:** Diagnosis will be confirmed with a CT scan. A subdural hematoma is a medical emergency and should be immediately referred to the emergency department.

Second Impact Syndrome

SIS results when a second blow to the head occurs before the symptoms associated with the first event have cleared. Following the initial concussion, brain cells survive in a vulnerable state.[4] If an athlete prematurely returns to sport and suffers a second impact, a disruption of the brain's autoregulatory system will lead to an increased intracranial vasodilation and pressure, resulting in mortality rates near 50% and morbidity rates of 100%.[4,5] Almost all reported cases of SIS have occurred in athletes under the age of 18.[4,6,7]

- **Onset:** The onset of symptoms can be observed within seconds to minutes following the trauma.

RED FLAG FOR DIAGNOSIS
Second Impact Syndrome

- Deterioration of cognition
- Rapid deterioration of posture and behavior
- Symptoms do not improve

- **Pain:** When evaluating pain, the athlete will have no response to pain, will have immediate loss of consciousness (LOC), and/or will be unresponsive.

- **Mechanism of injury:** The injury occurs by sustaining a hit or blow prior to the resolution of the initial head injury. SIS is associated with metabolic dysfunction and increasing intracranial pressure, which ultimately results in cerebral dysfunction.

- **Observation:** The athlete is noticeably motionless and demonstrates apparent loss of consciousness. No obvious swelling, deformity, or discoloration is commonly observed.

- **Palpation:** Not warranted.

- **Range of motion:** Not warranted.

- **Signs and symptoms:** If the athlete is conscious, symptoms begin with visual, motor, or sensory changes.[5] Within seconds to minutes, the athlete collapses with rapidly dilating pupils, loss of eye movement, and respiratory failure,[5] immediately after the second hit.

- **Neurological testing:** Evaluation should be limited to hasten transportation to the emergency department. If possible, primary neurologic examination should focus on pupils and reflexes. If time permits and patient is able, complete an upper quarter screen and cranial nerve evaluation.

- **Special tests:** None are currently available.

- **Diagnosis:** This diagnosis will be confirmed with CT or magnetic resonance imaging (MRI) and is a medical emergency. Once this differential diagnosis is suspected, stop everything, immediately activate emergency medical services, and transport the athlete to the emergency department as quickly as possible.

Skull Fracture

Skull fractures occur when direct and blunt forces are applied to the skull. The prevalence of skull fractures is higher in athletes who do not wear protective equipment compared to those who do. Skull fractures are typically classified into the following 3 categories:

1. Linear—Linear fractures are commonly referred to as *hairline fractures* and result in minimal movement on the skull bones. There may be localized swelling that results in a bump over the fracture site.

2. Comminuted—Comminuted fractures result in fragmentation of skull bones. The nature of the skull anatomy prevents comminuted fractures from movement away from the fracture site.

3. Depressed—Depressed fractures result when the force of the trauma causes an indentation. With depressed fractures, clinicians should be concerned about the possibility of fractured pieces of bone lacerating the meninges and brain.

- **Onset:** The onset of pain and symptoms for a skull fracture will occur acutely after the trauma.

RED FLAG FOR DIAGNOSIS
Skull Fracture

- Battle signs or raccoon eyes
- Positive halo test

- **Pain:** Pain will be reported as tender to palpation over the spot of trauma. Athlete may report headache stemming from trauma.

- **Mechanism of injury:** Blunt trauma to the head due to the skull being struck by a moving object or the skull striking a stationary object.

- **Observation:** The force required to fracture the skull often leads to a laceration of the covering scalp. Clinician should look for bruising or ecchymosis behind the mastoid process (battle signs) and around the eyes (raccoon eyes). Also look for leakage of cerebral spinal fluid or blood from the ear or nose. Look for bleeding from a laceration at the point of impact and/or loss of the rounded contour of the skull at the point of impact.

- **Palpation:** Firm but gentle palpation could reveal crepitus and deformation over the trauma location. Swelling may be palpated over the fracture site. Do not palpate areas that are obviously fractured or deformed.

- **Range of motion:** Do not continue evaluation if skull fracture is suspected. Range of motion is not warranted for this differential diagnosis.

- **Signs and symptoms:** The most common sign is pain over the point of impact. The athlete may experience headache, nausea, vomiting, and disorientation. Depending on the location of the fracture, cognitive deficits may be observed.

- **Neurological testing:** Upper and lower quarter screen and cranial nerve testing should be performed and will appear normal.

- **Special tests:** Halo test for leakage of cerebral spinal fluid can be conducted.

- **Diagnosis:** Diagnosis will be confirmed with x-rays. Since this is not able to be captured during the emergent period, transportation to the emergency department is warranted.

Generalized Seizure Disorder/ Epilepsy

A generalized seizure disorder is characterized by episodic, sudden involuntary contractions of a group of muscles resulting from excessive discharge of cerebral neurons. Generalized seizure disorder is also interchangeably called *epilepsy*. One percent of the population has seizures; 75% of new cases develop during childhood and adolescence.[3]

- **Onset:** The onset of active seizures will be acute; however, patients that have lived with this condition can recognize the onset of a seizure and chronic symptoms can be explained.

RED FLAG FOR DIAGNOSIS
Generalized Seizure Disorder

- ◉ Episodic seizures
- ◉ Unexplained periods of stupor

- **Pain:** Pain is typically not an indicator for this disorder.

- **Mechanism of injury:** Can be caused by systemic disease, head trauma, toxins, stroke, or hypoxic syndromes.

- **Observation:** Athlete may have LOC. Observe for posturing, bruising or ecchymosis behind the mastoid process (battle signs) and around the eyes (raccoon eyes), or cerebral spinal fluid leakage.

- **Palpation:** Areas will not be painful on palpation. There will not be evidence of deformity or crepitus. Palpation should be used to assess other differential diagnoses such as concussion or head trauma.

- **Range of motion:** Active, passive, and resistive range of motion will be within normal limits.

- **Signs and symptoms:** Behavior changes, alteration in consciousness, decreased sensation, and autonomic functioning may be present. Urinary and fecal incontinence may occur during seizures.

- **Neurological testing:** Upper quarter screen and cranial nerve testing should be performed and will appear normal.

- **Special tests:** Mini-mental status examination.

- **Diagnosis:** Diagnosis will be confirmed by electroencephalography (EEG). Once diagnosis is confirmed, most cases are managed well with medication. If active seizure occurs with an undiagnosed person, refer the patient to the emergency department. If diagnosis is present, manage the patient until the seizure resolves and the athlete returns to normal.

Ischemic or Hemorrhagic Stroke

A number of cerebrovascular diseases can be included within the differential diagnoses; however, ischemic and hemorrhagic stroke should be considered a potential diagnosis, as many of the symptoms are similar to those experienced during a head injury. Stroke remains one of the leading causes of death in the United States.[3] One-third of strokes are fatal, one-third leave some degree of permanent damage, and one-third have no long-lasting effects.[3] Ischemic strokes are caused by an interruption of blood flow in a cerebral vessel and are the most common type of stroke. Hemorrhagic strokes are caused by blood entering the brain tissue.[3] This type of stroke is typically caused by a blood vessel rupture from hypertension, aneurysm, or head injuries.

- **Onset:** The onset of pain and symptoms for a stroke will occur acutely.

RED FLAG FOR DIAGNOSIS
Ischemic or Hemorrhagic Stroke

- Dropping of facial structures
- Unilateral strength and sensation deficits

- **Pain:** Pain is traditionally reported as an increasing headache.

- **Mechanism of injury:** Ischemic or hemorrhagic stroke can be caused by aneurysm, trauma, erosion of vessels by tumors, or drug use.

- **Observation:** An athlete may present with unilateral drooping of facial structures, nystagmus of the eye, and/or dilated pupil. All signs will traditionally be unilateral in nature.

- **Palpation:** Palpation may reveal limited muscle tone. No evidence of swelling or crepitus will be found. Clinician should palpate all relevant bony, musculature structures.

- **Range of motion:** The athlete may present with limited to no active or resistive range of motion. Passive range of motion will be within normal limits.

- **Signs and symptoms:** Sudden feelings of weakness and unsteadiness, loss of movement in the arms or legs, numbness and/or tingling in any part of the body, excruciating headache, confusion, difficulty speaking, vomiting, blurred or double vision, or loss of vision in one eye can be observed.

- **Neurological testing:** Upper and lower quarter screen and cranial nerve testing should be performed and will be deficit on the affected side. Special emphasis should be placed on unilateral and bilateral strength testing.

- **Special tests:** Mini-mental status examination should be performed to establish cognitive function and obtain evidence for the possible areas of the brain affected.

- **Diagnosis:** Confirmed with CT. There is a window of treatment time that will improve the outcome for patients who have sustained a stroke. Quick referral and advanced life support will increase likelihood of survival with limited long-lasting effects.

Exertional Heat Illness

Exertional heat illness is an accumulation of body heat that results when the body's ability to cool itself is overwhelmed.[3] Exertional heat illness progresses through the following 3 stages:

1. Cramping—Heat cramps involve rapid water and electrolyte loss via perspiration.
2. Exhaustion—Heat exhaustion is the condition of near total body collapse. The body's heat control mechanism will remain intact, but will have difficulty dissipating heat.
3. Stroke—Heat stroke occurs when the body can no longer regulate and cool itself and reaches a temperature greater than 104°F. This condition causes significant cognitive dysfunction; hot, dry skin; and can lead to seizure, coma, or death. Previous history of heat illness increases the risk of sustaining heat illness again.

- **Onset:** The onset of symptoms for external heat illness is acute.

RED FLAG FOR DIAGNOSIS
Exertional Heat Illness

- Bilateral muscle cramping
- Syncope following exercise

- **Pain:** Distal cramping in the extremities is the primary pain report.

- **Mechanism of injury:** Overexposure to high temperatures and/or high humidity. The injury can also result from insufficient thermoregulatory control of the body and hypothalamus dysfunction.

- **Observation:** An athlete may appear red and sweating and may demonstrate increased respiration rate. Skin may be wet and red or hot and dry, depending on the condition.

- **Palpation:** Palpation may reveal increased muscle tone or spasm. Body may be hot to the touch and dry. Clinician should palpate all relevant bony and musculature structures. Patients will not report pain from palpation.

- **Range of motion:** Initially, the athlete may present with normal active, passive, and resistive range of motion. As the athlete progresses into heat stroke, range of motion will be limited due to muscle spasticity.

- **Signs and symptoms:** The patient may present with physical fatigue or dizziness, dehydration and/or electrolyte depletion, ataxia and coordination problems, increased heart rate and/or blood pressure, syncope, profuse sweating, pallor, headache, nausea, vomiting, diarrhea, cognitive dysfunction, blurred or double vision, stomach and/or intestinal cramps, persistent muscle cramps, and wet or dry skin (as patients move toward heat stroke, the body is unable to sweat and the skin will become dry).

- **Neurological testing:** Upper and lower quarter screen and cranial nerve testing should be performed and will appear normal.

- **Special tests:** Mini-mental status examination should be performed to establish cognitive function.

- **Diagnosis:** Confirmed with temperature readings. Most accurate temperature readings are obtained through rectal measures. Temperatures greater than 104°F signify heat stroke and are considered a medical emergency.

Concussion

This section provides the readers with a standard, brief synopsis of concussion injury for comparison in this chapter. Concussion evaluation will be covered in detail in Chapter 3.

- **Onset:** The onset of symptoms is typically acute; however, symptoms may appear 24 hours after a direct or indirect hit to the head.

RED FLAG FOR DIAGNOSIS
Concussion

◉ Individual variability; red flags not commonly used
◉ LOC and amnesia not required for diagnosis;
   are not red flags for concussion

- **Pain:** Pain is traditionally reported in the form of headache (around the location of the hit) or neck pain surrounding the trauma.

- **Mechanism of injury:** Injury can be caused by a blow to the skull or body that transmits jarring forces to the brain.

- **Observation:** Pupils should be examined for reactivity, accommodation, size, and nystagmus, but will appear normal. Ears and nose should be checked for bruising or ecchymosis behind the mastoid process (battle signs) and around the eyes (raccoon eyes) to rule out skull fracture. The athlete should be observed for posturing, which is indicative of a more severe neurological injury.

- **Palpation:** Clinician should palpate all relevant bony and musculature structures (specifically the facial bones, skull, temporal region, mastoid process, neck, and cervical spine) for crepitus, swelling, and deformity; temperature, however, will be normal.

- **Range of motion:** Active, passive, and resistive range of motion will typically be within normal limits; however, cervical spine movement may increase nausea if vestibular deficits are present.

- **Signs and symptoms:** Headache, dizziness, feeling in a "fog," feeling "slowed down," difficulty concentrating, sleepiness, nausea, vomiting, ringing in the ears (tinnitus), sensitivity to light/sound, blurred vision, irritability, balance difficulty, confusion, and amnesia (retrograde and anterograde).

- **Neurological testing:** Upper and lower quarter screen and cranial nerve testing should be performed and will appear normal.

- **Special tests:** Evaluation of memory, behavior, cognition, balance, eyes, vitals, motor function, and sensory function. Traditional tests include the Romberg test, Standardized Assessment of Concussion (SAC), Sports Concussion Assessment Tool 2 (SCAT2), traditional pencil-and-paper neuropsychological tests, computerized neuropsychological tests,

Balance Error Scoring System (BESS), tandem walking, and self-reported symptom checklist (see Chapter 3 for more detailed information on these special tests).

- **Diagnosis:** Confirmed with consistent objective findings from a multifaceted approach to testing and the presence of concussion-related symptoms.

Post-Concussion Syndrome

Post-concussion syndrome (PCS) results when cognitive impairments last for a period of time after the initial injury. The diagnosis of PCS is related to altered neurotransmitter function, but varies in the research regarding the necessary time to justify PCS (typically requires prolonged symptoms for greater than 3 months according to the *Diagnostic and Statistical Manual of Mental Disorders, Fourth Edition* [DSM-IV]).[8] McCrea et al[5] found that approximately 10% of subjects do not have symptom recovery at 10 days post-injury in adults. A small, though clinically significant group, perhaps as low as 5%, have persisting symptoms at 1 year.[9] Patients with a history of concussion, acute fatigue, physical illness, and orthopedic injury have demonstrated increased baseline self-reported symptom scores.[10] The nature of PCS and prolonged symptoms require clinicians to assess symptoms regularly and be aware of PCS.

- **Onset:** The onset of symptoms is typically chronic.

RED FLAG FOR DIAGNOSIS
Post-Concussion Syndrome

- Delayed cognitive decline
- Prolonged concussive symptoms

- **Pain:** Typically associated with headache.
- **Mechanism of injury:** Can be caused by the coup/contrecoup mechanism, rotation mechanism, or subconcussive trauma.
- **Observation:** The athlete may appear to be lethargic, have an altered level of consciousness, and/or be experiencing balance difficulties.

- **Palpation:** Palpation of appropriate structures includes all facial structures, nasal bone, occiput, orbit, musculature, throat, skull, and cervical spine. All palpations will appear normal.

- **Range of motion:** Active, passive, and resistive range of motion will be normal; however, the athlete may be unwilling to move body parts that disrupt equilibrium.

- **Signs and symptoms**

  ▷ **Early signs and symptoms:** Disorientation, confusion, headache, dizziness, blurred vision, nausea, drowsiness, and sleep disturbances.

  ▷ **Late signs and symptoms:** Decreased attention span, impaired memory, depression, sleep disturbances, headache, and trouble concentrating. Exercise may cause headaches, dizziness, and premature fatigue. Long-term deficits are balance and decreased cognitive performance.

- **Neurological testing:** Upper and lower quarter screen and cranial nerve testing should be performed and will appear normal.

- **Special tests:** Mini-mental status examination should be performed to establish cognitive function. Romberg, SAC/SCAT2, imaging, and neuropsychological testing can also be conducted. Symptom scale or checklist can be used for self-assessment.

- **Diagnosis:** Confirmed with neuropsychological testing and symptom checklist/scale for prolonged periods after concussive injury. As this is a diagnosis that is confirmed after symptoms do not resolve in a timely manner and the patient experiences additional emotional disturbances and cognitive decline, this diagnosis does not appear in isolation.

  Figure 2-1 shows a differential diagnosis concept map.

Summary

- Clinicians must work on developing differential diagnoses from the preliminary signs and symptoms.

- Differential diagnoses should provide guidance for the necessity of immediate or delayed referral processes.

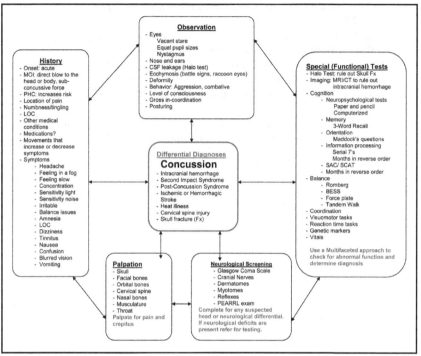

Figure 2-1. Concussion concept map.

- When in doubt, make sure the red flags for each diagnosis are examined and those diagnoses that are life threatening are triaged correctly.

- Clinicians should focus on performing a thorough yet efficient evaluation that successfully rules in and out relevant differential diagnoses.

References

1. Mueller FO. Catastrophic head injuries in high school and collegiate sports. *J Athl Train.* 2001;36(3):312-315.

2. McMinn R, Gaddum-Rosse P, Hutchings RT, Logan BM. *McMinn's Functional and Clinical Anatomy.* Barcelona: Mosby; 1995:193-213.

3. Seidel HM, Ball JW, Dains JE, Benedict GW. *Mosby's Guide to Physical Examination.* 4th ed. St. Louis, MO: Mosby; 1999.

4. McCrory PR, Berkovic SF. Second impact syndrome. *Neurology.* 1998;50:677-683.

5. McCrea M, Guskiewicz KM, Marshall SW, et al. Acute effects and recovery time following concussion in collegiate football players: the NCAA concussion study. *JAMA.* 2003;290(19):2556-2563.

6. Cantu R, Voy R. Second impact syndrome: a risk in any contact sport. *Phys Sports Med.* 1995;23:27-34.

7. Hunt TN. The psychometric properties of concussion assessment tools in high school athletics [dissertation]. Athens, GA: University of Georgia; 2006.

8. American Psychiatric Association. *Diagonstic and Statistical Manual of Mental Disorders.* 4th ed. Washington, DC; 1994:704-706.

9. Iverson GL. Outcome from mild traumatic brain injury. *Curr Opin Psychiatry.* 2005;18:301-317.

10. Piland SG, Ferrara MS, Macciocchi SN, Broglio SP, Gould TE. Investigation of baseline self-report concussion symptom scores. *J Athl Train.* 2010;45(3):273-278.

CONCUSSION EVALUATION ASSESSMENTS AND CLINICAL TOOLS

Evaluation is a critical skill for the clinician to develop in order to work effectively in his or her setting. Clinicians working within the sports medicine field have developed thorough and appropriate standardized and systematic approaches for the evaluation of musculoskeletal injuries. Clinicians take a thorough history to obtain specific physical signs and symptoms and can examine swelling, range of motion, joint laxity, muscle strength, functional tests, and noninvasive diagnostic tests. Based on the significant findings from these objective tests, clinicians can determine which structures are damaged and the severity of the injury. Obtaining the majority of this information provides a fairly accurate prognosis and clinicians can be confident that they have appropriately diagnosed the condition before beginning the appropriate management techniques.

Unfortunately, when clinicians begin evaluating a patient for concussion, the same standard, systematic process is not utilized. During concussion evaluation, clinicians perform a much more subjective evaluation. This evaluation begins with an incomplete history, fewer physical signs and symptoms, and less objective information that primarily revolves around eye movement, vision, balance, and coordination tests. The clinician may evaluate symptoms, memory, attention, and concentration, though that is not always the case. Due to the variability of each concussion and individual differences associated with the athlete him- or herself, there is less objective information and a more uncertain diagnosis, evaluation of injury severity, and less certain prognosis. The key to a good concussion evaluation requires a clinician to develop a systematic method, such as the one used to evaluate musculoskeletal injuries. All information should be collapsed into a working diagnosis. It is important to note that one piece of information is not more important than another piece, but should be examined in its entirety.

Recently, several agencies have produced position and consensus statements suggesting that clinicians employ a multifaceted approach to assessment and management of concussion.[1-4] Within the same statement, experts suggest obtaining baseline measures for concussion assessments. This is the

Hunt TN.
Cram Session in Evaluation of Sports Concussion:
A Handbook for Students & Clinicians (pp. 35-75).
© 2013 Taylor & Francis Group.

same idea as a preparticipation physical examination to understand what is present prior to any injury.

Baseline Testing

Baseline scores provide a quantitative starting point and allow for analysis of symptoms, neurocognitive issues, and motor changes following concussion. Completing a baseline assessment greatly enhances the sensitivity of each measure and allows for characterization of small concussion-related abnormalities that may otherwise go undetected.[5] Covassin et al[5] surveyed 399 certified athletic trainers and found that 95% use baseline testing.

When baseline measurements are not available, there are several ways to determine premorbid function. First, the use of age-appropriate normative data is suggested.[6] This approach has its limitations. The primary limitation is overlooking the subtle changes related to individual differences during concussion assessment when compared to age-dependent, industry-provided normative data. Second, normative data are only valid in the population for which they are obtained.[6-8] If the provided normative values are based on a population that is not representative of the individual being assessed, accurate interpretations in test performance following a concussive injury are difficult to impossible to determine.

When age-appropriate normative data are not appropriate or available, the clinician can obtain a premorbid picture from school and work records; personal documents; samples of work; creative performances; and descriptions from family, friends, and colleagues.[9] This approach has limitations as well. The first limitation is that the information obtained may only be a snapshot of the person.[9] Further, the amount of time required to gather and synthesize the information to only provide a rough estimate of premorbid performance may outweigh the usefulness of the information. This technique may be appropriate when the clinician is working with small populations of concussed athletes. Unfortunately, when no baseline tests are available, this time-consuming method may be the only option.

Implementation of baseline testing can be accomplished in several ways. The following guidelines are intended as a model, but the clinician will have to find out what works for him or her and the respective institution. For all methods, try to organize the plan prior to the start of the competitive season.

The first option is individualized testing. While individualized assessments provide vast information and a more intimate relationship with the patient, the number of clinicians necessary to complete one-on-one testing is unfortunately limited in many athletic settings. One-on-one testing is recommended to capture the subtlety of individual testing style, interpretation of the results, and the effort of the athlete. If the support staff to conduct one-on-one baseline testing is not available, mass testing can be a viable option.

Mass testing has become a widely utilized practice for concussion baseline testing in athletic settings. Within mass testing, clinicians should set up stations that will cover all elements. Each station should have at least 2 people trained in test administration. This can be accomplished during preparticipation physicals by adding additional stations within the examination room. Ideally, a clinician wants to perform baseline testing prior to the first session of contact or practice, as it could potentially result in an injury. This typically occurs during preseason training when athletes are acclimatizing to the weather and practice schedules. At this point, fatigue is less of a concern.

During mass testing, the following are recommended:

- Provide instructions in large group format.

- Provide enough space between athletes to avoid distraction. (For computerized testing, place athletes at every other computer.)

- Utilize technology for quick assessments of the population. There are new technological advances that decrease the amount of time necessary to conduct testing such as computerized neuropsychological testing, force plates, iPads (Apple, Cupertino, CA) and other tablets or smart phones to quickly administer and save testing information.

The individual variability of concussion and the effects of concussion on athletes suggest that multiple tools should be utilized to assess deficits that may be present following a concussive injury. The sports medicine team should agree on a standard multidimensional approach to concussion assessment. The most common concussion assessment battery begins with a good physical evaluation, imaging (if a fracture or hematoma is suspected), self-reported symptoms, and neuropsychological and postural testing. Including as much information as possible in the concussion evaluation provides the most comprehensive test battery for individualized concussion assessment. Additionally, findings from this encompassing battery produce more objective evidence to provide an accurate diagnosis and fairly decent prognosis. The recent addition of more advanced technological techniques to the concussion assessment battery enables the clinician to incorporate more information specific to areas most commonly injured following concussion.[1,2]

Technological advances will continue to add to concussion evaluation techniques. Trying to stay up-to-date on advancing technology can be a huge undertaking for a clinician. The key for concussion assessment is recognizing the tools available based on individual setting, population, and budget.

This chapter will focus on the traditional techniques associated with concussion evaluation. It will also introduce recent technology that can be utilized in concussion evaluation. While substantial evidence for new technology is limited, this chapter will provide as much evidence as is available for each tool and offer tips on how to incorporate these assessment tools into a step-by-step concussion evaluation process.

Traditionally, a traumatic event is witnessed or an athlete will come to the clinician with specific complaints. The process to determine differential diagnoses begins with witnessed or self-reported symptoms. That will be the first step in evaluation.

Self-Reported Symptoms

Self-reported symptoms are the most widely used tool for assessing concussions. Clinical symptoms reported by athletes are often the primary grounds on which a concussion is initially diagnosed. Approximately 85% of athletic trainers analyze symptoms as a means for concussion assessment.[10] During the course of an athletic season, most athletes will complain of some symptoms. The clinician must differentiate between normal symptoms, symptoms associated with the differential diagnoses discussed in Chapter 2, out-of-shape athletes, and concussion. Common symptoms associated with concussion include the following:

- Headache

- Dizziness

- Fatigue

- Feeling in a "fog"

- Feeling "slowed down"

- Difficulty concentrating

- Difficulty remembering

- Trouble falling asleep

- Sleeping more than usual

- Sleeping less than usual

- Nausea

- Vomiting

- Ringing in the ears (tinnitus)

- Sensitivity to light

- Sensitivity to sound

- Blurred vision

- Irritability

- Balance difficulty

- Sadness or feeling more emotional than usual

- Confusion

- Amnesia (retrograde and anterograde)

Piland et al[11] found that symptoms can be divided into 3 categories: cognitive, somatic, and physiological. The presence of symptoms is associated with neurophysiological changes that occur after brain injury. These symptoms are typically transient in nature and resolve in a timely fashion. Attention must be paid to concussion-related symptoms, such as headache, that occur naturally. Several investigators found that during baseline examination, athletes self-reported the presence of symptoms.[9,11,12] Awareness should be given to some of the symptoms that are also associated with other medical conditions, specifically heat illness. Clinicians may need to query commonly occurring symptoms such as headache, fatigue, and confusion to obtain a better understanding and limit differential diagnoses.

In 2010, more than 20 scales and checklists were utilized in athletics, clinics, and institutions for concussion assessment.[13] Unfortunately, many of the scales and checklists were found to have limited reliability and validity data and some symptom guidelines are not empirically based.[13-15] The symptom scale or checklist can take on many forms. Some symptom scales are based on Likert- or Guttman-type scales with descriptors of severity or duration, while others are designed using a yes or no format.

Many of the scales available to clinicians are derivatives of commonly utilized scales in concussion evaluation such as the Head Injury Scale (HIS), Graded Symptom Checklist (GSC) and Graded Symptom Scale (GSS), Rivermead Post-Concussion Symptom Questionnaire (RPCSQ), and Post-Concussion Scale (PCS).[16]

Head Injury Scale

The HIS scale focuses on somatic, cognitive, and physical symptoms commonly exhibited in concussive injury and includes severity and duration subscales.[17] The severity scale, a 7-point Likert scale, was used with anchors of 0 (not having the symptom) to 6 (severe symptoms). The duration scale was scored on a continuum from *never* to *always*. Three scores are obtained: duration, severity, and total score. Validity and reliability evidence has been obtained for assessment in both athletic and nonathletic samples.[13,17,18]

Graded Symptom Scale/Checklist

The GSS and the GSC are both derived from the HIS,[18] a theoretically-derived, self-report measure that has predominantly been used with adult athletes. The GSS consists of 16 items that are rated on Guttman-type scaling in terms of severity (0 = not having the symptom to 6 = severe symptom) and duration (number of days occurring during the week).[18]

On the GSC, symptoms are assessed by asking the patient to rate 20 items. Patients endorse whether they are experiencing the symptom that day and rate its severity on a 7-point Guttman scale (0 = not having the symptom to 6 = severe symptom).[17] The total symptom score and the total number of symptoms endorsed can be calculated.[18]

Rivermead Post-Concussion Symptom Questionnaire

The RPCSQ is a 16-item self-report measure.[19] Items on the RPCSQ were generated by reviewing commonly reported post-concussive symptoms in the literature.[19] Symptoms are rated as compared to "usual levels" to account for presence of pre-injury symptoms. The severity of symptoms are rated on a 5-point Guttman scale (0 = not having the symptom to 4 = severe symptom). A total score is calculated, as well as 3 subscales: cognitive, emotional, and somatic.[13,19]

Post-Concussion Scale

The PCS is a 22-item self-report measure.[20] Symptom items were chosen based on clinical experience with both professional and amateur athletes, with items worded to reflect the language of the players rather than medical terminology.[20] Symptoms are rated on a 7-point Guttman severity scale (0 = not having the symptom to 6 = severe symptom).

While self-reported symptoms are commonly utilized, the subjectivity of the report should always be questioned.[21] Covassin et al[5] found that no one should return a patient to participation while still symptomatic. Clinicians believe that self-reported symptoms are not reliable, as athletes subjectively report their symptoms and may be motivated to withhold symptom information to hasten their return to participation. Clinicians should utilize symptom reports along with objective evidence from the physical examination, cognitive tests, and balance tests to make the most accurate diagnosis and treatment plan.[1,3] Figure 3-1 provides a sample symptom checklist.

Based on symptom presentation, the clinician should proceed to the physical examination with the goal of ruling in or out each of the differential diagnoses.

Physical Examination

Physical examination is typically the most powerful piece of information for clinicians. It should follow the same evaluation process for a musculoskeletal evaluation. Physical examination typically occurs on the sideline or within the first few minutes of injury.

When surveyed in 2005, more than 95% of certified athletic trainers reported using the clinical examination as the primary assessment tool for concussion.[22] An increased percentage of certified athletic trainers utilizing physical examinations (up from 33%, as reported by Ferrara et al[10] in 1999) shows a trend for concussion awareness and assessment. Physicians appear to follow suit, as a recent study[23] of physician practice patterns found that physicians rely heavily on physical evaluation during the assessment process. Typical assessments in a physical evaluation include appropriate history; inspection; examination of nervous, motor, and sensory systems; and additional special tests. After the physical exam, a determination can be made and additional testing may be warranted.

History

During a physical evaluation, a complete history should be obtained. This provides information regarding the likelihood of previous concussion, symptoms occurring not related to the current concussive injury, or post-concussive symptoms. When a history is taken, the clinician should obtain as much information as possible to guide the evaluation to either rule-in or rule-out each diagnosis. History should include questions that are commonly asked with any musculoskeletal evaluation, along with questions specific to head injuries. General questions include how did it happen (mechanism of injury [MOI]); when did it happen; where (location of pain); and any previous history of injury. In addition to these general questions, specific questions associated with concussion should be included as well.

Post-Concussion Symptom Scale

Please tell us about the symptoms you are experiencing today. This is a list of symptoms that are commonly reported by individuals who have sustained a concussion. Use the scale below to describe which symptoms you are experiencing and the severity of the symptoms. If you do not have the symptom your score would be 0, if the symptom is severe your score would be 6.

Symptom Rating

None		Mild		Moderate		Severe
0	1	2	3	4	5	6

Symptom	
Headache	
Nausea	
Vomiting	
Balance problems	
Dizziness	
Fatigue	
Trouble falling asleep	
Sleeping more than usual	
Sleeping less than usual	
Drowsiness	
Sensitivity to light	
Sensitivity to noise	
Irritability	
Sadness	
Nervousness	
Feeling more emotional	
Numbness or tingling	
Feeling slowed down	
Feeling mentally foggy	
Difficulty concentrating	
Difficulty remembering	
Visual problems	
other	

Figure 3-1. Example of a symptom scale.

- **MOI:** Observing the incident or knowing how the injury happened provides clinicians with valuable information. If there was trauma, the location of trauma may produce focal deficits associated with local areas of the brain. For example, if the athlete fell backward and hit his or her head on the ground, the clinician might see a coup/contrecoup injury with damage to the occipital and frontal lobes that could result in deficits in information processing, decision making, and motor control.

- **Onset:** Concussion typically presents with an immediate onset of symptoms from the time of the trauma; however, symptoms can appear 24 hours after a direct or indirect hit to the head. Clinicians should obtain a detailed account of symptoms (such as nausea or vision difficulties) that were present prior to the injury, or symptoms that are now worse following the injury. Pre-existing symptoms can exacerbate concussion symptoms or provide a false sense of severity for the injury.

- **Previous history of injury:** Patients who have a previous history of concussion are 3 to 4 times more likely to sustain an additional concussion. There is evidence that concussed athletes are known to experience a second TBI within 1 year post-injury.[24,25] Furthermore, athletes with a previous history of concussion report more severe symptoms and demonstrate a prolonged recovery period. Other neurological conditions, such as Chiari malformation and learning disabilities, can further complicate the management and recovery from concussion.

- **Location of pain:** While pain is not a common symptom of concussion itself, clinicians may rely on the presence of headache (pain) in order to determine diagnosis. Location of the headache will provide information regarding the location of injury and deficits associated with the location of injury. For example, if the patient describes a headache in the occipital region, this may indicate damage to the occipital lobe and functional deficits may appear in motor coordination.

- **Complaints of numbness or tingling:** If numbness and/or tingling are present, the clinician should refer the patient to an emergency department to ensure there are not additional, more severe neurological conditions.

- **Presence of loss of consciousness:** Previously, loss of consciousness (LOC) was cited to be indicative of a more severe injury with longer recovery patterns. However, LOC is only seen in 8% of cases and current research no longer supports this theory.[26] The presence of LOC alone is not necessary for concussion diagnosis; however, if periods of LOC are present on-field, referral to the emergency department is warranted, especially in younger athletes with whom a more conservative approach is recommended.

- **History of other medical conditions:** Comorbid conditions may affect current symptoms. The clinician should determine if additional medical conditions make the patient susceptible to more concussions, delayed recovery, or affect management (eg, learning disability, psychiatric disorders, or history of migraine headache).

- **Recent medications taken:** Medications such as nonsteroidal anti-inflammatory drugs (NSAIDs), narcotics, and pain relievers may mask the presence of pain related to headache. Further, these medications may mask headache pain that is increasing. If possible, you do not want to mask symptoms with medication usage. Further, taking medications that increase blood flow would be contraindicated for a diagnosis or suspicion of an intracranial hematoma.

- **Movements or actions that increase or decrease symptoms:** Clinicians should ask about movements that increase or decrease the patient's symptoms of discomfort. An increase in symptoms with movement indicates deficits in the vestibular system. Patients may experience increased nausea and dizziness as a symptom of concussion with head movements.

Visual Inspection

Inspection of the athlete provides information prior to touching the patient or asking the patient a question. This inspection should start when the patient walks into the room or when the clinician walks toward the patient to start the examination.

Look to see if the athlete is in acute distress by asking the following questions:

- Does the athlete appear to be in pain?

- Does the athlete appear to have an altered gait or stumble?

During inspection, examine the following:

- **Presence of deformity:** Obvious deformity is typically not visible on the skull or brain. When obvious deformity is visible, there is a severe injury that warrants immediate referral to the emergency department.

- **Obvious visible lack of muscle tone or spasm:** This is indicative of trauma that has resulted in neurological involvement.

- **Discoloration:** Any traumatic force that may result in concussive injury has been applied with enough force to cause bruising and/or discoloration. If discoloration is present, the injury is not acute.

- **Ecchymosis:** Especially behind the mastoid process (battle signs) and around the eyes (raccoon eyes). This is indicative of severe bleeding and a skull fracture.

- **Position of the head and cervical vertebrae:** The head may be leaning toward one side or forward flexed. The positioning occurs to relieve stress on the muscles and/or ligaments.

- **Leakage of cerebral spinal fluid (CSF) from the nose and ears.**

- **Presence of posturing:** Posturing following head injury is associated with transient disruption of brain neurochemicals, which fades within seconds. There are 3 types of posturing associated with concussive injuries: decerebrate, decorticate, and flexion contracture.

  ▷ Decerebrate posturing presents with the head arched back, the arms down by the sides, and the legs straight.[27] The patient is rigid with teeth clenched.[28] The signs can be on just one side of the body or on both sides; it may be just in the arms and may be intermittent. Decerebrate posturing is usually indicative of more severe damage. It is exhibited by people with lesions or compression in the midbrain and lesions in the cerebellum.

  ▷ Decorticate posturing presents with the arms flexed or bent inward on the chest, the hands clenched into fists, the legs straight, and feet turned inward. Decorticate posturing indicates there may be damage to areas including the cerebral hemispheres, the internal capsule, and the thalamus.[19] It may also indicate damage to the midbrain and is indicative of a lesion above the brainstem.

  ▷ Flexion contracture presents with arms flexed across the chest in isolation. This is indicative of a spinal cord lesion at C5 to C6 level.

Inspection of the Eyes

The eyes are an essential part of the concussion evaluation. Anecdotally, many clinicians have seen the athlete with the glossy look during inspection. The eyes should be considered the direct link to the brain. A patient experiencing any problems with his or her eyes, visual acuity, and sight should be referred to a physician. Deficits and dysfunction of the eyes are traditionally associated with worse outcomes when head injuries are involved.

Each eye should be generally inspected. General inspection includes checking that pupils are equal, accommodating, and responsive and reactive to light (mnemonic: PEARRL). This inspection can be done with a pen light; however, if an ophthalmoscope is available, in addition to pupil reflexes, inspection of the optic nerve and retina can be accomplished.

Physicians should evaluate for the following:

- Size of the pupils

  ▷ Dilated pupils are indicative of a worse outcome or more severe symptoms. Dilated pupils are most commonly associated with an intracranial hematoma.

  ▷ Asymmetry of the pupils is indicative of a worse condition or more severe symptoms.

- Changes in iris color
- Changes in visual acuity
- Ability to focus on an object
- Vision can be assessed using a Snellen chart placed 20 feet from the patient. If a Snellen chart is not available, ask the patient if he or she can read something available to the clinician, such as the small line on the scoreboard or the writing on his or her shirt.
- Specific sight examinations should include the following:

  ▷ Peripheral vision

  ▷ Visual field

  ▷ Accommodation to light or darkness

  ▷ Color perception

- Eye tracking

  ▷ Eye tracking should be performed approximately 2 to 4 inches away going in all directions. The examiner should start at the center of vision and move away to each direction, always returning to the center of vision.

  ▷ During examination of eye tracking, the clinician should examine both the quantity and the quality of movement. Commonly, pain is seen in the extreme lateral and superior directions.

Palpation

- Palpation of appropriate structures includes all facial structures, nasal bone, occiput, orbit, musculature, throat, skull, and cervical spine.

- Palpation should evaluate crepitus, swelling, deformity, and temperature of the structures palpated.

Neurologic Evaluation

Neurological examination is vital in a concussion evaluation and should focus on determining the level of consciousness, orientation, dermatomes, myotomes, reflexes, and cranial nerves.

During evaluation of consciousness and orientation, clinicians should look for the quality and quantity of responses. The clinician should try to decipher normal and abnormal speed of response, clarity of the response, any speech difficulties, and/or overt confusion. These questions should be asked serially to determine if the patient's mental status is deteriorating.

Although it is common knowledge to refer to the emergency department when there is a decline in mental status, clinicians should be equally cautious if the patient is not getting better, as well. Traditionally, the clinician establishes whether the patient is responsive to verbal stimuli. The following section will highlight how to complete the neurological examination of a patient who is responsive to verbal stimuli. The evaluation should include examining the patient's pupillary reaction; upper and lower quarter screens which include the dermatomes, myotomes, and reflexes; and cranial nerves.

Pupillary Reaction to Light

- The clinician should cover the eye to try to establish a true contrast between light and dark.

- Have the athlete look straight ahead at a point past the examiner.

- Uncover the eye and then shine the light quickly into the pupil.

- The clinician should observe a quick reaction (constriction of the pupil) to the light.

- If the pupils are dilated, even after light is provided, this is indicative of an intracranial hematoma. If pupils are slow to constrict, the patient should be referred to a physician as this could be indicative of iritis, muscle strain, and/or a neurological condition.

Examine for Nystagmus

Nystagmus is involuntary contraction of the muscles around the eye that result in the appearance of the eye jumping during tracking. Nystagmus is indicative of a neurological response to injury.

Upper and Lower Quarter Screens

These neurological screens include dermatomes, myotomes, and reflexes. Upper and lower quarter screens should be performed any time the patient reports numbness or tingling and/or if there is a neurological condition in the differential diagnoses (inclusive of head injuries). Injuries to the spinal cord, such as laceration or complete rupture, result in complete dysfunction to any dermatome, myotome, or reflex below the level of injury. Injuries to individual nerves result in dysfunction of areas innervated by that specific nerve in isolation.

Dermatomes

Dermatomes are areas of skin innervated by one specific nerve. Dermatome assessment provides sensory information and should examine the following[29]:

- Superficial touch
- Superficial pain
- Vibratory response to tuning fork over joints or bony prominences on upper and lower extremities
- Evaluation of position sense with movements of the great toe or a finger
- Ability to identify familiar object by touch or manipulation
- Two-point discrimination
- Ability to identify letter or number drawn on palm of hand
- Ability to identify body area when touched

The clinician should ask the following questions:

- Can you feel me touching you?
- Does the body part feel the same on both sides?
- Can you discriminate between 2 points?

Do not ask, "Can you feel this?" as the athlete may be able to feel, but the feeling may be different; that would still be a positive finding.

Myotomes

Myotomes are a group of muscles that are innervated by one nerve. Myotome distributions of the upper and lower extremity are as follows[29]:

- C1/C2—neck flexion/extension

- C3—neck lateral flexion

- C4—shoulder elevation

- C5—shoulder abduction

- C6—elbow flexion/wrist extension

- C7—elbow extension/wrist flexion

- C8—thumb extension

- T1—finger abduction

- L2—hip flexion

- L3—knee extension

- L4—ankle dorsiflexion

- L5—great toe extension

- S1—ankle plantar-flexion

- S2—knee flexion

To check myotomes, the clinician should do break tests for each movement represented above. If the clinician obtains a positive neurological finding, the patient should be referred for additional testing to ensure no additional neurological conditions are present.

Reflexes

Reflexes should be evaluated using a reflex hammer. Clinicians should note the absence of reflexes, short or brisk reflexes, or delayed reflexes. The aforementioned reflex traits are indicative of a more serious neurological condition and should be referred for further assessment.[29] Common reflexes include the following:

- Biceps

- Brachioradialis

- Triceps

- Patella

- Achilles

- Babinski

- Homans'/Oppenheim

Cranial Nerves

Cranial nerves are nerves that arise from the brain, not the spinal cord. They are in pairs that innervate the ipsilateral side of the body. Cranial nerves can have sensory, motor, or a mixture of sensory and motor function.[29,30] Table 3-1 provides the name and function of each cranial nerve, with common mnemonics located in the table's footnote. Table 3-2 shows how each cranial nerve can be tested.

Neurological testing inclusive of cranial nerve assessment should be based on the presence of function. If a cranial nerve is not functioning, immediate referral to a physician is recommended. Neurological testing during concussion evaluation is typically normal. However, if the clinician finds abnormal neurological results, this may be indicative of a more severe injury and referral to a physician is warranted.

If the clinician is conducting the physical examination on the sideline or in the clinic acutely, additional quick screening tools (sideline assessments) are available to provide a screen of cognitive and balance function to aid in determining the diagnosis and whether referral to a specialist or emergency department is warranted.

Sideline Cognitive Assessment

Serial 7s

During the administration of serial 7s, the patient is asked to count backward from 100 by 7s (100, 93, 86, and so on). This test was intended to assess gross cognitive function and by itself cannot diagnose a particular illness. It is included in the mini-mental status examination and is used as a test of concentration and memory. However, the sensitivity of the test is not ideal for evaluation in isolation. Young et al[31] showed that 50% of high school athletes could not do serial 7s. Therefore, when possible, an objective test that can be documented appropriately should be utilized.

Table 3-1. Cranial Nerve Function

Number	Cranial Nerve[a]	Type	Function[b]
I	Olfactory	Sensory	Smell
II	Optic	Sensory	Vision
III	Oculomotor	Motor	Pupil reaction and size. Elevation of upper eyelid and eye abduction and downward rolling
IV	Trochlear	Motor	Upward eye movement
V	Trigeminal	Both	M: Muscles of mastication; S: Sensation to nose, forehead, temple, scalp, lips, tongue, and upper jaw
VI	Abducens	Motor	Lateral eye movement
VII	Facial	Both	M: Expression; S: Taste
VIII	Vestibulocochlear	Sensory	Hearing equilibrium
IX	Glossopharyngeal	Both	M: Pharyngeal muscles; S: Taste
X	Vagus	Both	M: Pharynx and larynx; S: Gag reflex
XI	Accessory	Motor	Trapezius and sternocleidomastoid (SCM) muscle function
XII	Hypoglossal	Motor	Tongue movement

M = Motor function; S = Sensory function

[a]Mnemonic device for the names of the cranial nerves: On Old Olympus Towering Tops A Fin And German Viewed Some Hops.

[b]Mnemonic device for the the function of the cranial nerves (ie, Sensory, Motor, or Both): Some Say Money Matters But My Brother Says Big Brains Matter Most.

Table 3-2. Cranial Nerve Testing

Function	Cranial Nerve	Clinical Test
Smelling	I	Based on self-report of smell, one nasal passage at a time with eyes closed
Eye assessment	II, III, IV, VI	Visual acuity, papillary reaction, and tracking
Facial expression	V, VII, X, XII	Smile, frown, swallow, stick out tongue
Balance	VIII	Romberg, BESS, standing
Speaking/hearing	VIII, IX, XII	Speaking to clinician, hearing the clinician
Shoulder shrug	XI	Resist shoulder girdle raise

BESS: Balanced Error Scoring System.

Three-Word Recall

Three-word recall is a clinical test of immediate memory, delayed memory, and recall. It is a condensed version of the traditional neuropsychological test (Hopkins Verbal Learning Test) that consists of a 15-word list. This is meant to be a gross screen of memory and recall abilities following head injuries.[32] This truncated version has demonstrated less sensitivity and specificity. During the administration of this exam, the patient is asked to remember 3 nonrelated words after a 10-minute delay. Selection of words should not be taken for granted. The clinician should strive for 2-syllable words in 3 different categories that are not related to each other or surrounding environmental cues.

Maddocks Questions

Maddocks questions are a set of questions developed to assess orientation and memory. This quick sideline tool should start with questions that happened most recently moving backward in time to end with questions that are furthest from the time of injury.[33] Maddocks questions are ideal for sideline orientation; however, they are not recommended for serial assessment beyond the acute assessment. Maddocks questions are typically scored as correct or not correct.[33]

The key to orientation questions is to make sure that the clinician knows the answers or someone is around who would know the correct answers. There are times when the patient will respond; however, the answer may be incorrect. It is just as important to note the speed, clarity, and quality of response as a right or wrong answer. If the clinician does not know the answer, he or she cannot properly evaluate the athlete.

Standardized Assessment of Concussion

The Standardized Assessment of Concussion (SAC) was developed by McCrea et al[34] in 2001 to be a quick, objective sideline screening tool of cognitive function. It was developed to be administered in 5 to 7 minutes, with sections that include orientation, immediate memory, concentration, and delayed recall.[35] The neurologic screen and exertional maneuvers are included on the SAC; however, they do not factor into the total score. These maneuvers can be a valuable source of information for clinical evaluation and initial diagnosis of concussion. Multiple forms (A through D) of the test are available to decrease practice and learning effects. The SAC has a maximum score of 30.[34]

Like other cognitive tools for concussion assessment, this tool is more useful if there are baseline scores. If baseline SAC scores for the patient were able to be obtained, a difference in 1 point is considered concussed. If baseline data are not available, normative values for high school and college athletes consider a total score of 25 to be average. Anything below a 25 would also be indicative of a concussed athlete.[34,35] This was not designed for and should not be used as a return-to-participation assessment tool. Scores on the SAC have been demonstrated to be reliable and valid for 48 hours after initial injury.[35-37] Technological advances have led to the development of a personal digital assistant (PDA) version of the SAC as well as an Apple application (Cupertino, CA).

The 6 SAC sections are as follows:

1. **Orientation:** Month, date, day of week, year, time.
2. **Immediate memory:** Word repetition. The key for this section is to complete the entire list and have the athlete repeat. These words should be given in 1-second increments.
3. **Concentration:** Reverse digits is a truncated version of digit span. Within the concentration section the patient is also required to state the months of year in reverse order.
4. **Delayed recall:** Once you complete the entire SAC, you determine the athletes' delayed recall by asking about the word list that was reviewed earlier. This should happen at the end of the test, approximately 5 minutes after immediate memory.
5. **Neurologic screening:** Pupils, recollection of the injury, strength, sensation, coordination.
6. **Exertional maneuvers:** 40-yard sprint, sit-ups, push-ups, and knee-bends.

Sport Concussion Assessment Tool

The original Sport Concussion Assessment Tool (SCAT) was developed as a clinical tool by experts in concussion during the Concussion in Sport Consensus Meeting held in Prague in 2005.[3] This tool was an evolution for SAC, and the group became more receptive to tools utilized during the initial on-field assessment. The original SCAT was further revised and enhanced during the second iteration (SCAT2) in 2009 and continued development in 2012.[3] The most current version is the SCAT3. This tool was developed to be a quick screen for on-field evaluation that includes commonly utilized tools to assess functions affected by concussion. These include memory, attention, symptoms, and balance. The development of the SCAT2 made the original SCAT obsolete. SCAT2 enables the calculation of the SAC score and Mattocks questions for sideline concussion assessment.[3,34-37]

The SCAT2 includes the following tools:

- Symptom scale
- Glasgow Coma scale (GCS)
- Maddocks questions
- SAC
- Balance examination—Modified Balance Error Scoring test
- Coordination examination—Finger-to-nose task

Directions for each section are provided, as well as sections for athlete information and concussion injury advice.

Currently, the SCAT2 is the cornerstone of most on-field assessment policies. This tool has been tested and can be utilized for athletes 10 years of age and older.[36] However, at the present time there are limited reliability and validity studies for the SCAT2.

Sideline Balance Testing

Two commonly utilized sideline balance tests are the Romberg test and the BESS.

Romberg Test

The Romberg test was commonly used to evaluate postural stability following an injury. The premise behind the Romberg test was to grossly evaluate somatosensory impairment by having the patient close his or her eyes to eliminate vision as a sensory source.[38-40] During the test, the patient is asked to stand on one leg, place the hands on the hips, and lean backward. The examiner is looking for gross balance dysfunction (primarily, the inability to perform the test).

Since the inception of the test, there have been various interpretations and modifications to increase the sensitivity and specificity for balance disorders. Several judgment criteria were established, such as the following:

- Time to first touch down
- Compensatory event[41,42]

Most modifications have occurred in foot position (stance) to alter the participant's base of support. However, each modification of the original Romberg test was criticized for the lack of sensitivity in situations where postural sway increases without the complete loss of postural stability in clinical populations, such as concussive injuries. Continued modification of the Romberg test resulted in the traditional BESS protocol.

Balance Error Scoring System

The BESS was developed as an objective assessment tool to be used by clinicians with minimal cost and training for the evaluation of postural stability following concussion.[43] It can be administered on the sideline with little equipment in a short period of time. During the test, the athlete stands on 2 surfaces (firm and foam) with eyes closed, performing 3 stances: double-leg stance, single-leg stance, and tandem (or heal-to-toe stance). The firm surface typically consists of the ground or a gymnasium floor. The foam surface traditionally consists of a 61-cm × 61-cm × 10-cm thick block of 0.88-kg density polyester open-cell foam (load deflection of 17.5 to 19.3, such as an Airex pad [Airex AG, Switzerland]). Each stance is held for 20 seconds with the subject's hands on hips and eyes closed. The total number of errors is calculated for each condition. Errors consist of the following:

- Opening eyes
- Stepping, stumbling, balance checks, or falling from the test position
- Moving hips into an angle greater than 30 degrees of flexion or abduction
- Lifting toes or heels from the test surface
- Remaining out of the test position for greater than 5 seconds.
- Taking hands off hips

Riemann found intertester reliabilities for each condition within the BESS compared to long force plate sway measures ranging from r = 0.78 to 0.96, dependent on the stance.[44] Moreover, BESS has been correlated to the Sensory Organization Test (SOT) composite scores and demonstrated similar recovery patterns.[43,44]

Considerable research has been conducted to examine the psychometric properties of BESS.[44-48] In studies following concussion, subjects exhibit acute postural stability alterations up to 5 days post-injury, with recovery usually occurring within 4 to 7 days post-injury compared to pre-injury baseline values.[43]

Although BESS and other postural measures appear to be sensitive to subtle deficits following concussion, there are several drawbacks. Administration of multiple trials of BESS results in practice effects, with the number of errors decreasing with each consecutive trial.[37] Further, the effects of fatigue increase the number of errors acutely, but athletes recovered after 20 minutes of rest following an exercise session.[36] Additional considerations, such as post-traumatic headache, have been demonstrated to increase balance deficits.[48]

Additional Sideline Assessments

King-Devick Test

Originally developed as a reading tool to assess the relationship between poor oculomotor functions and learning disabilities, it has been suggested as a screening tool to identify concussed patients. Poor oculomotor function has been associated with concussion.[49] The King-Devick (K-D) test asks athletes to read a series of charts of numbers that progressively become more difficult to read in a flowing manner.[49]

Longer times to completion are indicative of poor performance.[50] The K-D test is moderately correlated with the Military Acute Concussion Evaluation (MACE) (rs = -0.54; $P = 0.07$) for identification of concussion.[50] While there are limited studies[49,50] examining the K-D test, early pilot work appears that the K-D may be appropriate for use in identifying concussed individuals. Additional studies providing strong reliability and validity evidence are warranted before support of this test in all populations can be recommended.

Once a decision has been made that the differential diagnoses require activation of emergency medical services (EMS) or referral to the emergency department, several evaluation techniques come into play. If EMS is activated, having a common language when discussing level of consciousness is helpful and the GCS can be utilized.

Glasgow Coma Scale

The GCS is traditionally utilized among more severe brain-injured patients and typically does not provide significant information for clinicians conducting concussion evaluations. Most sport-related concussions do not register deficits on the GCS scale and thus would result in a perfect score (15) with no deficits.[51] However, it is beneficial to know the GCS as it can enhance communication between allied health care professionals, emergency medical technicians (EMTs), and emergency physicians, especially when activating EMS.

GCS provides a classification of injury based on the score obtained during testing. Scores are tallied as a total obtained for each additional level of consciousness.[51,52] Scores for GCS range from a minimum of 3 and a maximum of 15, where the higher the score, the milder the injury. Lower scores are indicative of a comatose state.

GCS provides a loose classification of head injuries. Three classifications are used: mild, moderate, and severe. GSC scores greater than 12 would be considered a mild head injury, while a score of 9 to 11 would indicate a moderate head injury. Any score less than 8 would be considered a severe head injury. The scale is based on the following 3 functions:

1. Best Eye Response (E)
   ▷ No eye opening = 1

   ▷ Eye opening in response to pain = 2

   ▷ Eye opening in response to speech = 3

   ▷ Eyes opening spontaneously = 4

2. Best verbal response (V)
   ▷ No verbal response = 1

   ▷ Incomprehensible sounds = 2

   ▷ Inappropriate words = 3

   ▷ Words expressing confusion = 4

   ▷ Oriented = 5

3. Best motor response (M)
   ▷ No motor response = 1

   ▷ Extension to pain = 2

   ▷ Abnormal flexion to pain = 3

   ▷ Flexion/withdrawal to pain = 4

   ▷ Localizes to pain = 5

   ▷ Obeys commands = 6

   Glasgow Coma score: E + V + M out of 15

Once the athlete arrives at the emergency department and/or physician's office, traditional imaging will be taken to rule-out a skull fracture or intracranial hematoma. However, if the clinician suspects a concussion in isolation, there is no need for imaging.

Imaging

The key to understanding the necessity for imaging during concussion assessment revolves around the nature of the injury. Concussion creates functional deficits rather than structural changes, and functional deficits cannot be observed using traditional imaging techniques.[2] At the Vienna meeting of the leaders in concussion assessment, it was reported[2] that imaging techniques such as x-ray, magnetic resonance imaging (MRI), and computerized topography (CT) would be unable to detect concussion unless there were gross structural changes in the brain.[2] CT and traditional MRI, therefore, may not be as useful as initially thought. Newer technologies may offer different techniques to evaluate brain function using imaging such as fMRI, SPECT, and ERP, which will be discussed in the following sections.

Upon arrival at the emergency department, most physicians will order x-rays and CT scans. X-rays will typically return with normal findings unless a skull fracture is present. The CT scan is the best test to evaluate and rule-out intracranial bleeding and other life-threatening vascular disorders.[53,54] Jagoda et al[55] found 3% to 10% of CT scans following concussion had a traumatic abnormality. Only 1% of those cases, however, required neurosurgical intervention.[55]

MRI constructs detailed anatomic images that are sensitive to traumatic lesions. MRIs are commonly utilized to identify soft-tissue injuries. MRI has been used acutely after injury, but concussed patients cannot be differentiated with MRI alone. Most abnormalities identified using MRI consisted of contusions and hematomas. The newest scans are magnetic source imaging (MSI), event-related brain potentials (ERP), positron emission tomography (PET), and functional MRI (fMRI).

Researchers are evaluating MRI spectroscopy studies following a concussive injury. Vagnozzi et al[56] imaged 40 concussed patients and 30 controls looking for N-acetylaspartate. This study found that it took 30 days for N-acetylaspartate to return to baseline in the concussed group and 45 days if it was a second concussion.[56] In addition, Vagnozzi et al[56] demonstrated that full metabolic recovery may take 1 month or more following injury. Wilde et al[57] examined MRI diffusion tensor imaging and observed detailed imaging of white matter tracts in the brain. The ability to use MRI to obtain detailed images of white matter may aid in examining subtle white matter changes in the brain following injury.[57] Newer technologies may offer different techniques to evaluate brain function using imaging.

fMRI may offer a more thorough assessment, as it provides information regarding neural function during task performance using a noninvasive technique.[58,59] This technique can be incorporated with the new dual task paradigms being researched in concussion assessment.[58] fMRI may be beneficial to measure recovery and brain compensation following concussion in adults.[58-60]

MSI is a new approach that includes the use of MRI to obtain anatomic information while investigating the electrophysiology data from magneto-encephalography (MEG).[61,62] MSI offers tracking of real-time brain activity, without distortion, by conduction through the brain, skull, and scalp.[63] ERP is another tool that can be used while performing working memory tasks, and may be a more sensitive measure of function.[52] ERP appears to be well suited in identifying cognitive dysfunction that may not be found with other neuropsychological testing.[63] For more complex concussive injuries, ERP used in combination with fMRI may be useful for complex cases.[64]

With the metabolic changes following concussion, utilization of PET and single-photon emission CT (SPECT) may provide more accurate information regarding the nature of the injury.[53,54,62] PET and SPECT can evaluate the metabolism of the specified region and blood flow, respectively, associated with activation of that region. These measures attempt to quantify correlations between metabolic flow and injury severity, post-concussion symptoms, and recovery.[63,64] Completed studies provide evidence that diffusion tensor imaging may be useful to identify subtle structural problems with concussion.[65] As technology continues to improve, clinicians' understanding of the effects and consequences of concussion should also improve.[66]

Grading Scales

Within the hospital setting, clinicians may utilize grading scales to communicate the severity of the injury to the patient, guardians, and/or other health care providers.

As of 2001, 25 published grading scales have been developed.[13,14,66] These grading scales are not based on empirical data but on the subjective opinions of physicians working with concussed athletes. The arbitrary recommendation of an athlete being asymptomatic for 7 days under rest and exertion has not been empirically justified. Common treatment and return-to-play guidelines, therefore, have been based purely on clinical experience.

Of the published grading scales and return-to-participation guidelines, 3 were most commonly used: Cantu,[67] Colorado,[68] and the American Academy of Neurology (AAN).[69] When surveyed, certified athletic trainers, on average, reported using the AAN more than any other grading scale.[10] These grading scales are typically based on several on-field markers such as loss of consciousness, post-traumatic amnesia, and/or concussion-related symptoms.

The review and analysis of grading scales has resulted in very little evidentiary support, which caused many grading scales to be eliminated in the literature or clinically at the time of injury. If utilized at all, clinicians suggest grading after the injured athlete has completely recovered because the treatment would be the same regardless of concussion grade. Thus in 2010, Dr. Robert Cantu[70] suggested that if grading were necessary or required, clinicians should assess the patient after he or she has completely recovered using time to recovery as a severity guideline. The inclusion of individualized care following concussion makes determining the severity of the injury important, from a research perspective, in determining long-term outcomes versus a clinical applicability regarding treatment. Clinically, the evidence for the GCS and grading scales is small and is no longer suggested in clinical care.[1] While removal of grading scales has been emphatically accepted, many clinicians still utilize grading scales when communicating with other health care professionals, patients, and patients' families. Until all clinicians have eliminated grading scales from clinical use, this topic must be discussed and understood.

Neurocognitive Assessment

After the initial visit to the emergency department, urgent care, or clinic, health care providers will request a follow-up appointment, at which time a more thorough evaluation will be conducted. Proper assessment of symptoms, cognitive, postural, and psychological assessment should be obtained. This in-depth assessment will aid in the management and education of concussion for the patient.

Once in a physician's or other clinician's office, an evaluation should occur that provides objective, specific information on appropriate diagnoses and a thorough understanding of the symptoms and potential underlying conditions. Neurologic symptoms are common in head injuries, but traditionally result with normal physical examination and imaging.[2] Further, brain function can be abnormal even when there is no obvious deformity, symptoms, or imaging. Conducting neurocognitive assessment can help clarify and objectify vague or seemingly minor complaints, uncover underlying symptoms (such as chronic headaches), and/or differentiate if the patient is not being truthful.

Sport Concussion Office Assessment Tool

As previously discussed, the SCAT2 was developed as a clinical tool by experts in concussion to be utilized as a quick and efficient sideline test. The simplicity and usefulness of this tool gained favor in clinical settings and it quickly became a cost-effective assessment that required little equipment to obtain valid objective information. However, the SCAT was created to be a quick sideline assessment tool and was not intended for serial administration or office utilization. Therefore, in 2010 a group of physicians modified the SCAT and developed the Sport Concussion Office Assessment Tool (SCOAT).[71]

The SCOAT was developed in South Africa as an adaptation from the SCAT2 to create a tool that can easily be implemented into an office or a clinical tool that can be administered serially.[71] Many of the modifications removed redundancies and added clinical features necessary for appropriate documentation. The key features that separate the SCOAT from the SCAT2 including the following:

- Removal of the GCS.

- Removal of Maddocks questions.

- Additional section to document general blood pressure, associated injuries, and neurological exam.

- Additional section to document prescribed management and compliance record.

- Additional section to document potential modifying factors for protracted recovery.

- Additional section to document neuroimaging.

- Additional section to document computerized cognitive testing.

- Change of the scoring to result in lower scores (with zero being optimal), resulting in better examinations.

Many of the changes implemented in the SCOAT were made due to clinical usefulness and ease. Sideline assessments are designed to be quick and efficient while gaining as much information as possible. In a clinical setting, however, more information and documentation is necessary for reimbursement and continuity of care.[71] In addition, more time is available to complete an evaluation. The SCOAT is a more comprehensive evaluation that includes items that would be utilized in a doctor's office while allowing the documentation of any serial and follow-up changes.[71] While this tool has not been validated and research has not yet been conducted using the tool, the SCOAT is currently used as a quick, clinical concussion assessment tool in an office (available online to the general public at www.sportsconcussion. co.za/Documents/SCOAT.pdf).

Though the SCOAT is the newest tool available for use in an office setting, the most common and widely used approach to concussion-related assessment has been to use a brief neurocognitive test battery. The neurocognitive test battery typically measures memory, cognitive processing speed, working memory, and/or executive function prior to and following a concussive injury.[66,72,73]

Neuropsychological testing has evolved from traditional pencil-and-paper testing to include computerized batteries such as Automated Neuropsychological Assessment Metrics (ANAM; Defense and Veterans Brain Injury Center, Washington, DC), CNS Vitals (CNS Vital Signs LLC, Morrisville, NC), Cogsport/Axon Sports (CogState Ltd, Victoria, Australia), Headminder Concussion Resolution Index (CRI; Headminder Inc, New York, NY), and Immediate Post Assessment of Concussion Tool (ImPACT; ImPACT Applications, Pittsburgh, PA) with many more being developed every year. Neuropsychological testing is used to provide a sensitive index of higher brain functioning by measuring memory, attention, and the speed of cognitive processing.[74] In sport-related concussion assessment, the most common approach has been to administer a brief battery of less than 40 minutes that measures functions usually affected by brain injury. These functions include memory, cognitive processing speed, working memory, and/or executive function.[73-76]

While neuropsychological testing has hit the forefront of concussion assessment, it is not the final or most complete method of testing. The type of platforms for neuropsychological tests utilized are specific to the institution in which they are used. Most neuropsychological tests, regardless of the platform, appear to capture the deficits observed in professional, collegiate, and high school research.[72-78]

The traditional pencil-and-paper tests have a robust history and normative data base for most populations involved in neuropsychological testing. These tests are time consuming, with the average pencil-and-paper neuropsychological battery taking 2 to 3 hours per patient to administer. Further, they require individualized testing and advanced training in neuropsychology to administer. Many of the tests are copyright protected, require permission to use, and come with hefty associated costs.

Computerized platforms boast a more sensitive and specific reaction time and information processing speed.[77-79] Computerized neuropsychological testing can measure within the millisecond. The platform is ideal for mass testing in an institution's computer lab. Further, normative data that are appropriate for each population are typically installed within the program. Research involving these computerized platforms is being published at exponential rates; however, the platforms can be expensive and the availability of evidence in multiple populations, especially those athletes with comorbidities such as low socioeconomic status or learning disabilities, is limited.[74,75,77,80-85]

Traditional pencil-and-paper and computerized neuropsychological platforms both have advantages and disadvantages. Either platform is a useful adjunct in the total evaluation process, but findings may be difficult to interpret without baseline data. No clinician or researcher would suggest that globally one platform is better than another. That decision should be made alongside the sports medicine team to obtain the best information available for the population. Additional research needs to be conducted to make solid clinical recommendations as clinicians may need to examine other factors and testing during the evaluation of concussion.

Balance Assessment

Postural stability, or balance assessment, has been recognized as an important piece of the concussion assessment battery.[42,43,86,87] The construct of postural stability is composed of the postural control system. The postural control system uses 3 sensory systems to operate a feedback control circuit between the brain and the musculoskeletal system.[42] Under normal circumstances, postural stability is maintained by integrating the somatosensory, visual, and vestibular systems. If one system is not operating correctly, the other systems should be able to compensate.[42,86]

Typically, what is seen following a concussion is that the athlete will have difficulty integrating information from the 3 components of the balance mechanism. While the somatosensory aspect appears to remain normal, integration between the visual and vestibular components does not function properly.[88] At this point, patients will rely heavily on one aspect of balance integration (typically visual).

The balance assessment may be more sensitive to neurocognitive changes following injury than some pencil-and-paper tests. Thompson et al[89] found postural deficits following injury after symptom resolution. Guskiewicz et al[88] found deficits in postural stability when cognitive deficits dissipated. Deficits in posturography, with no deficits in other domains, suggests the balance mechanism operates on a different pathway in the brain.[90,91] Broglio et al[92] found that self-reported symptoms of balance problems correlated with balance testing (rs = 0.57). This moderate correlation supports continued use of self-reported symptoms in addition to balance testing. Resch et al[93] found that a balance task plus cognitive task may isolate subtle mental processes that can be used in concussed college athletes. These studies establish the need for a multifaceted approach to assessment specific to various areas of brain functioning. Posturography provides the clinician with valuable information in making a return to participation decision.

There are multiple tools to assess balance in a clinic setting. While the Romberg test and BESS balance tests are used to determine gross balance deficits, additional balance tests performed on force platforms can be utilized. These force platforms cost thousands of dollars.[94] Force platforms are utilized to obtain postural sway and center of gravity measures. More comprehensive units can determine motion across individual joints.[92-95] Commercially available force platforms utilize balance stances and tests on technologically advanced platforms to obtain more sensitive measures of center of gravity; postural stability; and medial, lateral, anterior, and posterior sway.

The gold standard for postural stability is the Smart Balance Master SOT (NeuroCom International Inc, Clackamas, OR) developed by Nashner. The Smart Balance Master is a computerized force platform. The SOT consists of 3 trials of 6 conditions (18 total trials), with each trial lasting 20 seconds. The test systematically alters visual and somatosensory referencing in an attempt to individually evaluate the 3 components of the balance mechanism (visual, vestibular, and somatosensory). The SOT is the gold standard for postural stability in concussion; however, the SOT is not portable and is very expensive. The SOT has been able to distinguish clinical populations as displayed by lower results in at least 1 of the 6 conditions.[96] Further, the SOT has test-retest and intraclass reliabilities of 0.66 and 0.57, respectively.[41,44,96] The SOT has demonstrated deficits following concussion and is sensitive to the condition.[41,44,92-95]

The Clinical Test of Sensory Interaction of Balance (CTSIB; Balance Master 6.0 [NeuroCom]) is a timed test that was developed for systematically testing the influence of the visual, vestibular, and somatosensory input of standing balance. The CTSIB consists of 3 conditions: eyes opened, eyes closed, and the use of a visual conflict dome.[40] This test can be performed on the floor, which makes it inexpensive, effective, and easily applicable to most populations. For each condition the amount of time spent in the stance and amount of body sway is utilized to assess balance. The test has been found reliable in youth, young adults, and populations with vestibular conditions.[40] The Biosway Force Platform (Biodex Medical Systems, Shirley, NY) utilizes the CTSIB on a force platform and obtains postural stability as well as postural sway measures.

Additional Clinical Tools

The push for a multifaceted approach to concussion assessment has led to the development of tests not traditionally examined in concussed athletes. This approach is suggested to enhance the sensitivity and validity of all findings; experts have recommended a combination of tests including cognitive, motor, reaction time, postural, visuomotor, and self-reported symptoms. New tests are arriving on the market constantly to help clinicians become more effective and efficient in assessing multiple aspects of concussion. Many of these tests are meant to be cost- and time-effective.

Nintendo Wii Fit Balance Board

The use of the Nintendo Wii (Redmond, WA) gaming system is becoming more popular and widespread in therapy for varying populations. There appear to be many practical advantages of utilizing the force platform such as decreased amount of time, space, amount of equipment necessary, and increased cost efficiency.[97-101]

The Wii Fit Balance Board has 4 force plates under each foot of the board. The force plates quantify the vertical and horizontal forces exerted on them by each foot via strain gauges that measure the anterior/posterior center of vertical force position.[98] Clark et al[97] found that the center of pressure scores from the Wii Fit Balance Board had good to excellent test-retest reliability when utilizing a custom software package. However, when custom software is not available, the Wii Fit appears to have poor concurrent validity, intrasession, and intersession reliability.[99] While the Wii Fit is cost-effective, evidence does not support the reliability of these measurements.[98-101] The tool is currently being assessed with the utilization of customized computer programming and additional research needs to be conducted to determine the reliability, validity, and clinical applicability of using this module in concussion assessment.

Visuomotor Pointing Task

Researchers in Waterloo, Ontario, Canada, developed a Visuomotor Pointing Task designed to induce a speed-accuracy trade-off to measure motor planning and execution performance in concussed athletes.[102] Athletes are asked to point as quickly and accurately as possible to the target when it appears after a randomized delay. Athletes complete 40 trials (10 per target size) with each hand.[102] Decreases in performance speed were indicative of concussion, not changes in speed-accuracy trade-offs. The Visuomotor Pointing Task was compared to a computerized neuropsychological platform and the motor task may be better able to detect long-term effects of concussion.[102] Very few studies have been performed utilizing this tool and, as such, experts cannot suggest this in use with multiple populations until additional research on validity and reliability can be conducted.[102]

Clinical Reaction Time Measure

Researchers at the University of Michigan developed a clinical reaction time (RTclin) measure designed to be utilized quickly in any setting.[103] The RTclin was measured using a measuring stick embedded in a weighted rubber disk.[103] The athlete sits with a forearm resting on a horizontal desk or table surface with the hand positioned at the edge of the surface. The athlete holds the hand sufficiently open to fit around, but not to touch, the weighted disk portion of the clinical reaction time apparatus.[103] The examiner drops the tool at randomized intervals and the athlete is asked to catch the tool as quickly as possible. Fall distance is measured from the most superior aspect of the athlete's hand after catching the device. This tool has demonstrated test-retest reliability over successive seasons.[104] One-year reliability is correlated to a computerized reaction time test and test-retest intraclass correlation coefficients have been estimated as 0.645.[103] Long-term reliability has been supported with research. However, limited evidence is available to establish the validity of preseason baseline to post-injury comparisons.[104]

Genetic Markers

Researchers have begun to examine genetic markers in concussion assessment to determine the occurrence of a concussive injury as well as an individual's susceptibility and predictive recovery.[105,106] The most commonly reported biomarkers have been S100B, apolipoprotein epsilon 4 allele (ApoE-4), and Alpha II spectrin breakdown proteins (SBDP).[106] Interpretation of the genetic information requires researchers to obtain genetic markers during baseline assessment and then serially acutely after the injury. Unfortunately, these methods are expensive, time consuming, genetically invasive, and not appropriate for all clinicians working with athletes.

S100B

S100B has been well established as a neurobiochemical marker of structural brain damage and correlates well with severity of injury.[107-109] Researchers have investigated S100B serum levels to examine elevation of S100B acutely following concussive injury. It appears elevation of this marker is short lived. For this reason, several papers focused on the use of biochemical markers to detect and define the severity of brain damage and predict outcome after traumatic head injury with mixed results.[109]

ApoE-4

There are mixed results in determining the usefulness of ApoE-4 in discovering patients' susceptibility to a concussive injury.[110] Some studies suggest no association between carrying the ApoE-4 allele and sustaining a concussion.[111,112] However, it appears that there is a relationship between ApoE-4 and a history of concussion.[110] Carriers of all 3 ApoE rare (or minor) alleles were nearly 10 times more likely to report a previous concussion and may be at a greater risk of concussion than noncarriers.[111] Promoter minor allele carriers were 8.4 times more likely to report multiple concussions and may be at a greater risk of multiple concussions compared to noncarriers. Further, college athletes with an ApoE promoter G-219T TT genotype may be at increased risk for having a history of concussions, especially more severe concussions.[112]

Alpha II Spectrin Breakdown Proteins

Examination of SBDP in cerebral spinal fluid appears to predict injury severity and mortality after TBI and may be a useful complement to the clinical assessment.[113,114] Elevation of calpain- and caspase-specific SBDPs is a significant finding in patients with TBI, indicating that intact brain spectrin and SBDP levels are closely associated with the specific neurochemical processes evoked by severe TBI.[115] Unfortunately, data have been confirmed in severe brain injury and consistent findings in concussive injuries have not been elucidated.

Currently, there is not sufficient high-level evidence to recommend genetic testing as a clinical measure due to the ambiguity of the current research findings. The preliminary findings of genetic testing support the need for additional prospective studies to identify the relationship to concussive injuries and ensure the appropriate use of genetic testing in concussion assessment.

Although this chapter provided details of concussion assessment tools, it is not all-inclusive. It is recommended that concussion assessment tools should be utilized in combination to obtain the most complete information regarding deficits post-concussion. Broglio and colleagues[92] found that neuropsychological testing in combination with self-reported symptoms produced a sensitivity of 89% to 96% following concussion. Since deficits following concussion carry the same variability as the individuals who sustain concussions, a multifaceted approach provides information regarding as many deficit areas as possible.

After concluding the evaluation, the clinician should examine all of the information they have obtained in order to make a diagnosis. The more objective information a clinician can gather, the more the clinician can trust the diagnosis and develop a fairly accurate prognosis. Figure 3-2 shows an evaluation flow chart that illustrates these common steps.

Summary

- A standardized concussion evaluation process that everyone within the sports medicine team can agree on should be developed.

- Concussion evaluation should be multifaceted and incorporate as much objective information as possible.

- Baseline test patients when possible in order to identify the subtle deficits following concussion.

- Due to the individual differences of the athlete and resultant concussive deficits, clinicians should perform multiple tests to assess any deficits that may occur following a concussive injury.

- Numerous tools exist; however, to date, abundant high-level evidence is unavailable for most.

- Concussion assessment should be specific to the population, age, gender, training of the examiner, space, and time constraints.

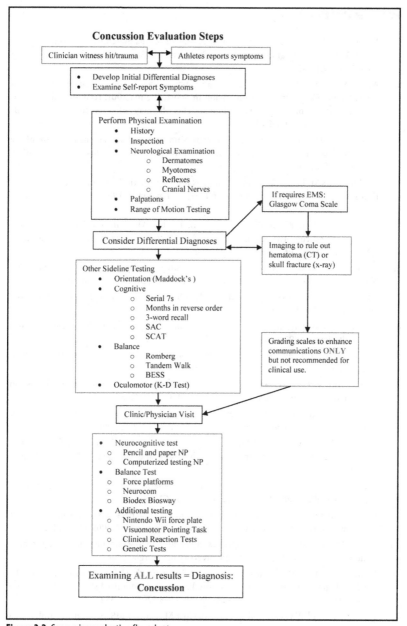

Figure 3-2. Concussion evaluation flow chart.

References

1.   McCrory P, Meeuwisse W, Johnston K, et al. Consensus Statement on Concussion in Sport, 3rd International Conference on Concussion in Sport, Zurich 2008. *Clin J Sport Med.* 2009;19:185-200.

2.   Aubry M, Cantu R, Dvorak J, et al. Summary and agreement statement of the First International Conference on Concussion in Sport, Vienna 2001: recommendations for the improvement of safety and health of athletes who may suffer concussive injuries. *Br J Sports Med.* 2002;36(1):6-10.

3.   McCrory P, Johnston K, Meeuwisse W, et al. Summary and agreement statement of the 2nd International Conference on Concussion in Sport, Prague 2004. *Br J Sports Med.* 2005;39(4):196-204.

4.   Guskiewicz KM, Bruce SL, Cantu R, et al. National Athletic Trainers' Association position statement: management of sport-related concussion. *J Athl Train.* 2004;39(3):280-297.

5.   Covassin T, Elbin RJ, Stiller-Ostrowski JL, Kontos AP. Immediate post-concussion assessment and cognitive testing (ImPACT) practices of sports medicine professionals. *J Athl Train.* 2009;44:639-644.

6.   Spreen O, Strauss E. *A Compendium of Neuropsychological Tests: Administration, Norms, and Commentary.* 2nd ed. New York: Oxford University Press; 1998.

7.   Baumgartner TA, Jackson AS, Mahar MT, et al. *Measurement for Evaluation.* Boston: McGraw-Hill; 2003:96-119.

8.   Spreen O, Risser A, Edgell D. *Developmental Neuropsychology.* New York: Oxford University Press; 1995:37-77.

9.   Parker RS. *Concussive Brain Trauma: Neurobehavioral Impairment and Maladaption.* Boca Raton, FL: CRC Press Incorporated; 2001.

10.   Ferrara MS, McCrea M, Peterson CL, et al. A survey of practice patterns in concussion assessment and management. *J Athl Train.* 2001;36:145-149.

11.   Piland SG, Motl RW, Ferrara MS, et al. Evidence for the factorial and construct validity of a self-report concussion symptoms scale. *J Athl Train.* 2003;38:104-112.

12.   Field M, Collins MW, Lovell MR, et al. Does age play a role in recovery from sports-related concussion? A comparison of high school and collegiate athletes. *J Pediatr.* 2003;142(5):546-553.

13.   Alla S, Sullivan SJ, McCrory P. Defining asymptomatic status following sports concussion: fact or fallacy? *Br J Sports Med.* 2012;46(8):562-569.

14.   Alla S, Sullivan SJ, Hale L, McCrory P. Self-report scales/checklists for the measurement of concussion symptoms: a systematic review. *Br J Sports Med.* 2009;43(suppl):i3-i12.

15.   Hunt TN. The psychometric properties of concussion assessment tools in high school athletics [dissertation]. Athens, GA: University of Georgia; 2006.

16.   Downs SH, Black N. The feasibility of creating a checklist for the assessment of the methodological quality both of randomised and non-randomised studies of health care interventions. *J Epidemiol Community Health.* 1998;52(6):377-384.

17.   Piland SG, Motl RW, Guskiewicz KM, McCrea M, Ferrara MS. Structural validity of a self-report concussion related symptom scale. *Med Sci Sports Exer.* 2006;38:27-32.

18.   Mailer BJ, Valovich McLeod TC, Bay RCB. Healthy youth are reliable in reporting symptoms on a graded symptom scale. *J Sport Rehabil.* 2008;16:11-20.

19. King NS, Crawford S, Wenden FJ, Moss NE, Wade DT. The Rivermead Post Concussion Symptoms Questionnaire: a measure of symptoms commonly experienced after head injury and its reliability. *J Neurology.* 1996;242:587-592.

20. Wrightson P, Gronwall D. *Mild Head Injury: A Guide to Management.* New York: Oxford University Press; 1999.

21. Gagnon I, Swaine B, Friedman D, Forget R. Exploring children's self-efficacy related to physical activity performance after mild traumatic brain injury. *J Head Trauma Rehabil.* 2005;20:436-439.

22. Notebaert AJ, Guskiewicz KM. Current trends in athletic training practice for concussion assessment and management. *J Athl Train.* 2005;40(4):320-325.

23. Hunt TN, Trombley A. Physician management of sport-related concussion at the collegiate level. *Athl Train Sports Health Care.* 2010;2:227-234.

24. Kushner D. Mild traumatic brain injury toward understanding manifestations and treatment. *Arch Intern Med.* 1998;158(15):1617-1624.

25. Randolph C. Implementation of neuropsychological testing models for the high school, collegiate and professional sport setting. *J Athl Train.* 2001;36(3):288-296.

26. Oliaro S, Anderson S, Hooker D. Management of cerebral concussion in sports: the athletic trainer's perspective. *J Athl Train.* 2001;36(3)257-262.

27. Register-Mihalik J, Guskiewicz KM, Mann JD, Shields EW. The effects of headache on clinical measures of neurocognitive function. *Clin J Sports Med.* 2007;17:282-288.

28. Ayling J. Managing head injuries. *Emerg Med Serv.* 2002;31(8):42.

29. Magee DJ. *Orthopaedic Physical Assessment.* 4th ed. St. Louis: Elsevier; 2006:1-181.

30. McMinn R, Gaddum-Rosse P, Hutchings RT, Logan BM. *McMinn's Functional and Clinical Anatomy.* Barcelona: Mosby; 1995:193-213.

31. Young CC, Jacobs BA, Clavette K, Mark DH, Guse CE. Serial sevens: not the most effective test of mental status in high school athletes. *Clin J Sport Med.* 1997;7(3):196-198.

32. Cullum CM, Thompson LL, Smernoff EN. Three-word recall as a measure of memory. *J Clin Exp Neuropsychol.* 1993;15(2):321-329.

33. Maddocks DL, Dicker GD, Saling MM. The assessment of orientation following concussion in athletes. *Clin J Sport Med.* 1995;5(1):32-35.

34. McCrea M, Randolph C, Kelly J. *Standardized Assessment of Concussion: Manual for Administration, Scoring and Interpretation.* Waukesha, WI.

35. McCrea M. Standardized mental status testing of acute concussion. *Clin J Sport Med.* 2001;11:176-181.

36. McCrea M, Kelly J, Randolph C, et al. Standardized assessment of concussion (SAC): on site mental status evaluation of the athlete. *J Head Trauma Rehab.* 1998;13:27-36.

37. McCrea M, Kelly JP, Kluge J, Ackley B, Randolph C. Standardized assessment of concussion in football players. *Neurology.* 1997;48(3):586-588.

38. Jinguji TM, Bompadre V, Harmon KG, et al. Sport concussion assessment tool–2: baseline values for high school athletes. *Br J Sports Med.* 2012;46(5):365-370.

39. Black FO, Wall C, Rockette HE, Kitch R. Normal subject postural sway during the Rhomberg test. *Am J Otolaryngol.* 1982;3:309-318.

40. Cohen J, Blatchly C, Gombash L. A study of the clinical test of sensory interaction and balance. *Phys Ther.* 1993;73:346-354.

41. Riemann BL, Guskiewicz KM. Assessment of mild head injury using measures of balance and cognition: a case study. *J Sport Rehabil.* 1999;6:283-289.

42. Jansen ER, Larsen R, Olsen. Quantitative Romberg's test. Measurement and computer calculation of postural stability. *Acta Neurol Scand.* 1982;66:93-99.

43. Guskiewicz KM, Riemann BL, Perrin DH, Nashner LM. Alternative approaches to the assessment of mild head injury in athletes. *Med Sci Sports Exer.* 1997;29(7 suppl):S213-S221.

44. Riemann BL, Guskiewicz KM. Effects of mild head injury on postural stability as measured through clinical balance testing. *J Athl Train.* 2000;35(1):19-25.

45. Susco TM, Valovich McLeod TC, Gansneder BM, Shultz SJ. Balance recovers within 20 minutes after exertion as measured by the balance error scoring system. *J Athl Train.* 2004;39(3):241-246.

46. Valovich TC, Perrin DH, Gansneder BM. Repeat administration elicits a practice effect with the Balance Error Scoring System but not with the Standardized Assessment of Concussion in high school athletes. *J Athl Train.* 2003;38(1):51-56.

47. Valovich-McLeod T, Perrin DH, Guskiewicz KM, Shultz, SJ, Diamond R, Gansneder BM. Serial administration of clinical concussion assessments and learning effects in healthy young adults. *Clin J Sports Med.* 2004;14(5):287-295.

48. Register-Mihalik JK, Mihalik JP, Guskiewicz KM. Balance deficits after sports-related concussion in individuals reporting posttraumatic headache. *Neurosurgery.* 2008;63:76-80.

49. King D, Clark T, Gissane C. Use of a rapid visual screening tool for the assessment of concussion in amateur rugby league: a pilot study. *J Neurol Sci.* 2012;320(1-2):16-21.

50. Galetta KM, Brandes LE, Maki K, et al. The King–Devick test and sports-related concussion: study of a rapid visual screening tool in a collegiate cohort. *J Neurol Sci.* 2011;309(1):34-39.

51. Gómez PA, Lobato RD, Ortega JM, De La Cruz J. Mild head injury: differences in prognosis among patients with a Glasgow Coma Scale score of 13 to 15 and analysis of factors associated with abnormal CT findings. *Br J Neurosurg.* 1996;10(5):453-460.

52. Jones C. Glasgow Coma Scale. *Am J Nurs.* 1979;79(9):1551-1557.

53. Bazarian JJ, Blyth B, Cimpello L. Bench to bedside: evidence for brain injury after concussion—looking beyond the computed tomography scan. *Acad Emerg Med.* 2006;13:199-214.

54. Mendez CV, Hurley RA, Lassonde M, Zhang L, Taber KH. Mild traumatic brain injury: neuroimaging of sports-related concussion. *J Neuropsychiatry Clin Neurosci.* 2005;17(3):297-303.

55. Jagoda AA, Cantrill SV, Wears RL. Clinical policy: neuroimaging and decision-making in adult mild traumatic brain injury in the acute setting. *Ann Emerg Med.* 2002;40:231-249.

56. Vagnozzi R, Signoretti S, Cristofori L, et al. Assessment of metabolic brain damage and recovery following mild traumatic brain injury: a multicentre, proton magnetic resonance spectroscopic study in concussed patients. *Brain.* 2010;133(11):3232-3242.

57. Wilde EA, McCauley SR, Hunter JV, et al. Diffusion tensor imaging of acute mild traumatic brain injury in adolescents. *Neurology.* 2008;70:948-955.

58. Broglio SP, Tomporowski PD, Ferrara MS. Balance performance with a cognitive task: a dual task testing paradigm. *Med Sci Sports Exer.* 2005;37(4):689-695.

59. Lovell MR, Pardini JE, Welling J, et al. Functional brain abnormalities are related to clinical recovery and time to return-to-play in athletes. *Neurosurgery.* 2007;61(2):352-360.

60. Chen JK, Johnston KM, Petrides M, Ptito A. Recovery from mild head injury in sports: evidence from serial functional magnetic resonance imaging studies in male athletes. *Clin J Sport Med.* 2008;18:241-247.

61. McAllister TW, Sparling MB, Flashman LA, Saykin AJ. Neuroimaging findings in mild traumatic brain injury. *J Clin Exp Neuropsychol.* 2001;23(6):775-791.

62. Theriault M, De Beaumont L, Trembley S, Lassonde M, Jolicoeur P. Cumulative effects of concussions in athletes revealed by electrophysiological abnormalities on visual working memory. *J Clin Exp Neuropsychol.* 2011;33(1):30-41.

63. Broglio SP, Moore RD, Hillman CH. A history of sport-related concussion on event-related brain potential correlates of cognition. *Int J Psychophysiol.* 2011;82(1):16-23.

64. Gosselin N, Saluja RS, Chen JK, Boattari C, Johnston K, Ptito A. Brain functions after sports-related concussion: insights from event-related potentials and functional MRI. *Phys Sports Med.* 2010;38(3):27-37.

65. Cubon VA, Putukian M, Boyer C, Dettwiler A. A diffusion tensor imaging study on the white matter skeleton in individuals with sports-related concussion. *J Neurotrauma.* 2011;28(2):189-201.

66. Johnston KM, McCrory P, Mohtadi N. Evidence-based review of sport-related concussion: clinical science. *Clin J Sport Med.* 2001;11:150-159.

67. Cantu R. Posttraumatic retrograde and anterograde amnesia: pathophysiology and implications in grading and safe return to play. *J Ath Train.* 2001;36(3):244-248.

68. Colorado Medical Society. *Report of the Sports Medicine Committee: Guidelines for the Management of Concussion in Sports.* Denver; Colorado Medical Society. 1991

69. American Academy of Neurology. Practice parameter: the management of concussion in sports. *Neurology.* 1997;48:581-585.

70. Cantu R, Hyman M. *Concussion and Our Kids Place.* Houghton Mifflin Harcourt; 2012.

71. Patricios J, Collins R, Branfield A, Roberts C, Kohler R. The sports concussion note: should SCAT become SCOAT? *Br J Sports Med.* 2012;46(3):198-201.

72. Lovell MR, Iverson GL, Collins MW, McKeag D, Maroon JC. Does loss of consciousness predict neuropsychological decrements after concussion? *Clin J Sport Med.* 1999;9(4):193-198.

73. Macciocchi SN, Barth JT, Alves W, Rimel RW, Jane JA. Neuropsychological functioning and recovery after mild head injury in collegiate athletes. *Neurosurgery.* 1999;39(3):510-514.

74. Lau BC, Collins MW, Lovell MR. Sensitivity and specificity of subacute computerized neurocognitive testing and symptom evaluation in predicting outcomes after sports-related concussion. *Am J Sports Med.* 2011;39(6):1209-1216.

75. Pellman EJ, Lovell MR, Viano DC, Casson IR, Tucker AM. Concussion in professional football: neuropsychological testing—part 6. *Neurosurgery.* 2004;55(6):1290-1303.

76. Barth J, Alves W, Ryan T, et al. Mild head injury in sports: neuropsychological sequelae and recovery of function. In: Levin H, Eisenber H, Benton A, eds. *Mild Head Injury.* New York, NY: Oxford University Press; 1989:257-275.

77. Lovell MR, Collins MW, Iverson GL, et al. Recovery from mild concussion in high school athletes. *Neurosurgery.* 2001;98(2):296-301.

78. Comper P, Hutchinson M, Magrys S, Mainwaring L, Richards D. Evaluating the methodological quality of sports neuropsychology concussion research: a systematic review. *Brain Inj.* 2010;24(11):1257-1271.

79. Collie A, Maruff P, Darby DG, McStephen M. The effects of practice on the cognitive test performance of neurologically normal individuals assessed at brief test-retest intervals. *J Int Neuropsychol Soc.* 2003;9(3):419-428.

80. Echemendia RJ, Bruce JM, Bailey CM, Sanders JF, Arnett P, Vargas G. The utility of post-concussion neuropsychological data in identifying cognitive change following sports-related MTBI in the absence of baseline data. *Clin Neuropsychol.* 2012;26(7):1077-1091.

81. Erdal K. Neuropsychological testing for sports-related concussion: how athletes can sandbag their baseline testing without detection. *Arch Clin Neuropsychol.* 2012;27(5):473-479.

82. Covassin T, Elbin RJ, Harris W, Parker T, Kontos A. The role of age and sex in symptoms, neurocognitive performance, and postural stability in athletes after concussion. *Am J Sports Med.* 2012;40(6):1303-1312.

83. Kontos AP, Dolese A, Elbin RJ, Covassin T, Warren BL. Relationship of soccer heading to computerized neurocognitive performance and symptoms among female and male youth soccer players. *Brain Inj.* 2011;25(12):1234-1241.

84. Lange RT, Iverson GL, Franzen MD. Neuropsychological functioning following complicated vs. uncomplicated mild traumatic brain injury. *Brain Inj.* 2009;23(2):83-91.

85. Gualtieri CT, Johnson LG. Computerized test battery sensitive to mild and severe brain injury. *C Medscape J Med.* 2008;10(4):90.

86. Ingersoll CD, Armstrong CW. The effects of closed-head injury on postural sway. *Med Sci Sports Exer.* 1992;24(7):739-743.

87. Guskiewicz KM, Perrin DH. Research and clinical applications of assessing balance. *J Sport Rehabil.* 1996;5:45-63.

88. Guskiewicz KM, Ross SE, Marshall SW. Postural stability and neuropsychological deficits after concussion in collegiate athletes. *J Athl Train.* 2001;36(3):263-273.

89. Thompson J, Sebastianelli W, Slobounov S. EEG and postural correlates of mild traumatic brain injury in athletes. *Neurosci Lett.* 2005;377:158-163.

90. Guskiewicz KM, Perrin DH. Effect of mild head injury on cognition and postural stability [abstract]. *J Athl Train.* 1998;33(suppl):S1-S8.

91. Shumway-Cook A, Horak F. Assessing the influence of sensory interaction on balance. *Phys Ther.* 1986;66:1548-1550.

92. Broglio SP, Sosnoff JJ, Ferrara MS. The relationship of athlete-reported concussion symptoms and objective measures of neurocognitive function and postural control. *Clin J Sport Med.* 2009;19(5):377-382.

93. Resch JE, May B, Tomporowski PD, Ferrara MS. Balance performance with a cognitive task: a continuation of the dual-task testing paradigm. *J Athl Train.* 2011;46(2):170-175.

94. Chaudhry H, Bukiet B, Ji Z, Findley T. Measurement of balance in computer posturography: comparison of methods. A brief review. *J Bodyw Mov Ther.* 2011;15(1):82-91.

95. Mondell EM, Furman JM, Herdman SJ, Konrad HR, Shepard NT. Computerized dynamic platform posturography. *Otolaryngol Head Neck Surg.* 1997;117(4):394-398.

96. Kaye J, Panzer VP, Camicioli R. Balance in the healthy elderly: posturography and clinical assessment. *Arch Neurol.* 1997;54(8):976-981.

97. Clark RA, Bryant AL, Pua Y, McCrory P, Bennell K, Hunt M. Validity and reliability of the Nintendo Wii balance board for assessment of standing balance. *Gait Posture.* 2010;31(3):307-310.

98. Bekter AL, Desai A, Nett C, Kapadia N, Szturm T. Game-based exercises for dynamic short-sitting balance rehabilitation of people with chronic spinal cord and traumatic brain injuries. *Phys Ther.* 2007;87(10):1389-1398.

99. Hirsch MA, Toole T, Maitland CG, Rider RA. The effects of balance training and high-intensity resistance training on persons with idiopathic Parkinson's disease. *Arch Phys Med Rehabil.* 2003;84(8):1109-1117.

100. Barin K. Dynamic posturography: analysis of error in force plate measurement of postural sway. *IEEE Engineering in Medicine & Biology Magazine.* 1992;11(4):52-56.

101. Wikstom EA. Validity and reliability of Nintendo Wii Fit Balance Scores. *J Athl Train.* 2012;47(3):306-313.

102. Locklin J, Bunn L, Roy E, Danckert J. Measuring deficits in visually guided action post-concussion. *Sports Med.* 2010;40(3):183-187.

103. Eckner JT, Kutcher JS, Richardson JK. Between-seasons test retest reliability of clinically measured reaction time in National Collegiate Athletic Association division I athletes. *J Athl Train.* 2011;46(4):409-414.

104. Eckner JT, Kutcher JS, Richardson JK. Effect of concussion on clinically measured reaction time in 9 NCAA division I collegiate athletes: a preliminary study. *PM R.* 2011;3(3):212-218.

105. Finnoff JT, Jelsing EJ, Smith J. Biomarkers, genetics, and risk factors for concussion. *PM R.* 2011;3(10 suppl 2):S452–S459.

106. Ingebrigtsen T, Romner B. Biochemical serum markers of traumatic brain injury. *J Trauma.* 2002;52(4):798-808.

107. Elovic E, Edgardo B, Cuccurullo S. Traumatic brain injury. In: Cuccurullo SJ, ed. *Physical Medicine and Rehabilitation Board Review.* Demos Medical; 2004:54-55.

108. Filippidis AS, Papadopoulos DC, Kapsalaki EZ, Fountas KN. Role of the S100B serum biomarker in the treatment of children suffering from mild traumatic brain injury. *Neurosurg Focus.* 2010;29(5):E2.

109. Piazza O, Storti MP, Cotena S, et al. S100B is not a reliable prognostic index in paediatric TBI. *Pediatr Neurosurg.* 2007;43(4):258-264.

110. Kristman VL, Tator CH, Kreiger N, et al. Does the apolipoprotein epsilon 4 allele predispose varsity athletes to concussion? A prospective cohort study. *Clin J Sport Med.* 2008;18(4):322-328.

111. Tierney RT, Mansell JL, Higgins M, et al. Apolipoprotein E genotype and concussion in college athletes. *Clin J Sport Med.* 2010;20(6):464-468.

112. Terrell TR, Bostick RM, Abramson R, et al. APOE, APOE promoter, and Tau genotypes and risk for concussion in college athletes. *Clin J Sport Med.* 2008;18(1):10-17.

113. Mondello S, Robicsek SA, Gabrielli A, et al. αII-spectrin breakdown products (SBDPs): diagnosis and outcome in severe traumatic brain injury patients. *J Neurotrauma.* 2010;27(7):1203-1213.

114. Cardali S, Maugeri R. Detection of alphaII-spectrin and breakdown products in humans after severe traumatic brain injury. *J Neurosurg Sci.* 2006;50(2):25-31.

115. Farkas O, Polgár B, Szekeres-Barthó J, Dóczi T, Povlishock JT, Büki A. Spectrin breakdown products in the cerebrospinal fluid in severe head injury-preliminary observations. *Acta Neurochir.* 2005;147(8):855-861.

4

MANAGEMENT AND RECOVERY OF SPORT-RELATED CONCUSSION

Historically, the management technique used for severe traumatic brain injury consisted of cognitive rehabilitation and occupational and physical therapy progressing through each stage of recovery while monitoring the healing process.[1] The 6 stages of recovery following severe head injury are marked by the goal to return the patient to premorbid function.[1] The cognitive rehabilitation and occupational and physical therapy used in severe traumatic brain injury (TBI) is, unfortunately, not appropriate for concussions. During the acute recovery period following concussion, clinicians may not recognize neurological or cognitive dysfunction due to adrenaline, fear, or somatic trauma. Therefore, clinicians have historically implemented a "wait and see" approach with daily, weekly or biweekly monitoring until the patient gets better on his or her own.

The focus for most clinicians regarding the medical management of sports-related concussion has been that the majority (80% to 90%) of concussive injuries resolve in 7 to 10 days.[2] This recovery period has been demonstrated to take longer in children, adolescents, and other populations such as athletes with a previous history of injury, learning disability, lower socioeconomic status, psychological conditions, and/or individuals who encounter barriers to recovery.

Clinicians strive to provide the best clinical management for recovery from concussion, but there are situations when appropriate management strategies fail. Understanding the barriers to success is crucial.[1] When these barriers are not addressed, recovery will be prolonged and secondary injuries may occur. The most common barriers include the following:

- Inaccurate prognosis
- Inappropriate therapy
- Family resistance and/or lack of support
- Failure to utilize behavior modifications
- Impatience

Hunt TN.
*Cram Session in Evaluation of Sports Concussion:
A Handbook for Students & Clinicians* (pp. 77-91).
© 2013 Taylor & Francis Group.

These barriers should be addressed during the initial visit and consultation with the team involved in the patient's management and recovery. Educating the athlete and support staff on the management plan and why/how it was developed will strengthen support from those involved and ease implementation of the plan.

Due to the individual variability of injury and recovery, most experts support the convention that everyone deserves individualized management. Further, recovery will vary based on the following factors:

- Prognostic factors (history, comorbidities)

- Advice given to athlete

- Athlete's willingness/ability to follow advice

No specific medical therapies are currently available for sports-related concussion and treatment options available for those suffering from concussion symptoms are limited. Most patients improve with education, cognitive rest, and time for the brain to recover. This chapter will provide details regarding the current management techniques of cognitive rest, pharmacological interventions, and modifiers affecting concussion recovery.

Cognitive Rest

The cornerstone of sports-related concussion management is physical and cognitive rest until symptoms resolve and then a graded program of exertion prior to medical clearance and return to participation.[2-4] Very little is published on the notion of cognitive rest. This time should allow the athlete to rest the brain and should be treated similarly to putting an athlete on crutches for an ankle sprain. Cognitive rest within the treatment protocol requires patients to disengage from academic, physical, and social activities.

During the first few days of recovery following an injury, it is important to emphasize to the athlete that physical and cognitive rest is required. Activities that require physical exertion, concentration, and attention may exacerbate the symptoms and delay recovery.

The goal of cognitive rest is to return the balance between energy available and energy needs.[5] Therefore it is encouraged to use the brain as little as possible for activities of daily living. This is applied to activities in and out of school. Academically, this may require scholastic accommodations (which will be discussed in detail in Chapter 6). The athlete should not engage in exertional physical activity before beginning the structured and supervised return-to-participation progression. Excessive post-injury activity may adversely affect recovery.[6] Social and home-based activities are currently limited during the acute phase of recovery. These include social networking practices, such as text messaging, Facebook (Facebook Inc, Melo Park, CA) activity, television watching, and video gaming.[2] Basically, the rest period should last as long as symptoms are the greatest and should be in place until the athlete can return to activities of daily living without significant symptom increase.

Very few studies have been conducted examining cognitive rest. Majerske and colleagues[6] found that high levels of overall activity may interfere with recovery, whereas more moderate levels may be acceptable, or even beneficial. Moser et al[7] examined high school and collegiate athletes after 1 week of cognitive rest and found decreased symptom reporting and improvement of cognitive test scores measured by the Immediate Post Assessment of Concussion Tool (ImPACT). The preliminary data suggest that a period of cognitive and physical rest may be a useful means of treating concussion-related symptoms, whether applied soon after a concussion or weeks to months later.[7] However, there are no randomized control trials to accurately account for normal recovery as measured through controls.

Pharmacological Support

Currently there are no medications approved in the United States specifically for concussions. There are, however, some pharmacological treatments that provide relief for specific concussion symptoms.[7-17] Very few well-designed studies have examined medications for concussion. To date, there is no evidence that medications speed recovery. While most experts believe that pharmacological support may help with symptoms, such as sleep disturbance and headache, true recovery is identified as being symptom free at rest/exertion without the aid of medications.

Clinicians believe that pharmacologic treatment should only be implemented in the following 2 specific circumstances[9]:

1. Management of specific symptoms (eg, sleep disturbance, anxiety, and nausea).
2. To modify the underlying pathophysiology of the condition with the aim of shortening the duration of the concussion symptoms.[9]

Recommendations for pharmacologic therapies should only be considered and provided by health care professionals with training and experience in managing concussion.[9] Throughout the history of therapeutic treatment, many pharmacologic options have been suggested for all grades of brain injury. However, most of the research is being conducted on patients with severe brain injuries and is not directly applicable to concussion.[8,9]

Several classifications of drugs have demonstrated at least moderate efficacy for symptoms related to concussive injuries.

Nicotinamide (Vitamin B3)

Nicotinamide (vitamin B3) is an organic compound and has been proven to be a powerful neuroprotectant when given to animals who have sustained a brain injury.[10-12] When vitamin B3 is administered to rats after they had head injuries, strong evidence suggests that it can improve functional recovery.[12] While the evidence is strong within the animal models, the literature is scarce in humans and translation of findings is limited.

Amitriptyline

Amitriptyline is a tricyclic antidepressant and has been studied specifically for treating post-traumatic headaches with some mixed results.[14,15] It appears it may be effective in doses of 75 to 225 milligrams per deciliters (mg/d),[15] whereas a more rigorous clinical trial[16] found no benefit for amitriptyline. In a retrospective review of 23 patients treated with amitriptyline for headaches after sustaining a head injury,[14] 90% made an excellent or good recovery. However, not all investigations have seen such an effect.[15]

Omega-3

Docosahexaenoic acid (DHA) is an omega-3 fatty acid that is a primary structural component of the human brain, cerebral cortex, sperm, testicles, and retina. DHA has demonstrated a protective effect against the biochemical brain damage that occurs after a traumatic injury in rats.[17] Rats that were given DHA prior to an induced brain injury demonstrated smaller increases in 2 key markers for brain damage (amyloid precursor protein [APP] and caspase-3), as compared to controls.[18] DHA may provide prophylactic benefit to the brain against traumatic injury; however, direct translation to human studies is warranted.[18]

Hyperbaric Chambers

The use of hyperbaric oxygen (HBO_2) therapy as a medical treatment to support and accelerate the body's own healing mechanisms to speed recovery from injury, surgery, or chronic illness has been well established.[19] These mechanisms include improved glucose metabolism, reduction of cerebral edema, and cerebral vasoconstriction.[19] Researchers have applied low-pressure HBO_2 therapy protocols to additional chronic cerebral disorder cases.[19-26] There is mounting evidence for HBO_2 therapy as a means to both accelerate and improve recovery among patients suffering from sport-related concussion.[24,25] Wright et al[1] found that delivering hyperbaric oxygen to soldiers after improvised explosive device-induced concussion produced rapid improvement of symptoms.[26]

The following medications have been investigated with little to no evidence to support use in concussive injuries[27-30]:

- Nonsteroidal anti-inflammatory drugs (NSAIDs)

- Corticosteroids

- Free radical scavengers or antioxidants

- Calcium channel antagonists

Currently, management strategies are geared around suppression of concussion-related signs and symptoms. When concussive symptoms resolve in a traditional time period, additional management is not typically warranted. In cases in which prolonged symptoms are present, referral to additional therapists may be warranted. The most common referrals are for physical therapy to treat vestibular and postural deficits, speech therapy to treat language deficits, and neuropsychologists to treat cognitive retraining. Based on symptom and deficit presentation, additional referrals may be given. Pharmaceutical choice for a patient depends on the symptom characteristics, and each decision should be made on an individual case-by-case basis. Well-designed randomized control trials regarding medical management options for concussive injuries need to be conducted before use of any treatment for all populations is recommended.

Recovery Following Concussion

Return to participation is based on the complete recovery from concussion. But how do clinicians know if an athlete is completely recovered? That is the question that many clinicians ask following a concussive injury. No one conclusive test has been able to determine that an athlete is ready to return to participation. The best clinical practice has been to wait until the patient is asymptomatic, to make sure all objective tests have returned to normal (or as normal as can be determined without baseline data), and to rely on population-based research to determine the best estimate. Clinicians have tried to provide rough guidelines for recovery length; however, there are several modifiers that will prolong recovery from the injury. These modifiers or comorbidities include neurological, stress induced, constitutional, psychological, and medical factors that can exacerbate symptoms and create deficits in neuropsychological test scores.[31] This section will discuss recovery and modifiers that may prolong recovery.

Age

The primary modifier of recovery is age. Generally speaking, the younger the athlete is at the time of injury, the longer the recovery.[32] The developing brains of children and adolescents are thought to respond differently than those of adults following concussive injury. Recovery following brain injury depends on the severity of the injury, age at injury, and the developmental period during which the concussion occurred.[32-34]

On average, college athletes will recover in 7 days though recovery could be as early as 48 hours.[35-41] Researchers have found that 90% of college football players experience symptom resolution within 7 days.[42,43] However, 10% to 14% of college athletes experienced prolonged recovery following concussion. High school athletes on average recover in 14 to 17 days and report an increase in symptoms when compared to collegiate athletes following concussion.[35,44-47] However, Covassin and Elbin[48] examined neuropsychological test scores to track cognitive performance following injury and found high school athletes may need up to 21 days to recover.

Age-appropriate assessment and management tools should be utilized to ensure that athletes are not deemed recovered prematurely. Junior high school athletes will recover in 21 to 24 days; those aged younger than 10 years may take 4 weeks or more.[43] Cognitive immaturity and metabolic differences in younger athletes has been suggested as a reason for greater dysfunction and slowed recovery.[49] Giza and Hovda[50] found in animal models that immature brains were 60 times more sensitive to glutamine. Unfortunately, there is little research available focusing on concussion in athletes who are junior high school age and younger. These recovery times are anecdotal based upon low-level evidence and clinician experience.

Currently, there is little research and few cognitive/postural tests available for youth participants (aged younger than 9 years). There are a limited number of pencil-and-paper tests available in youth versions, and these traditional tests can be time consuming. Instead, clinicians and researchers must take into account the development and growth process during maturation. Typically, these neuropsychological test batteries are composed of downward extensions of tests used in adult populations.[34,51] Some of these tests may not be appropriate because the domains being tested might require different demands on the child's cognitive system.[51] This gap in the literature and test batteries is currently understood and several projects are in process to provide pediatric versions of commonly utilized batteries.

Improper Management

The inability to adequately rest the brain has also been suggested to pro-long recovery. In animals, researchers have found a period of brain vulnera-bility that lasts for 7 days following injury. Premature return to participation and emotional stress add significant demands on cognitive function, espe-cially on information-processing skills.[52] Activity, both mental and physical, has been found to increase symptoms and delay recovery. Many clinicians anecdotally suggest rest for at least 48 hours after injury.[50,53] However, ani-mal models suggest a period of vulnerability that lasts 7 to 10 days after the injury.[50] The effects of a subsequent injury appear greatest during the first week following the injury.[53]

The effect of increased physical exertion, while still suffering from con-cussion, has been studied in both animal and human models.[52] In animal models, rats with concussions that were forced to exercise had an increase in brain cell death, which led to prolonged recovery.[54] If exercise was delayed 1 week post-injury, recovery appeared more complete.[50,54]

There is an apparent benefit to exercise if properly timed. Uninjured animals demonstrated increased brain growth factors when allowed to voluntarily exercise.[54] These findings were duplicated in humans where excessive post-injury activity adversely affected recovery. Majerske et al[6] found that both high-level and no activity prolonged recovery, while mod-erate activity was best. Moreover, the risk for second impact syndrome (as described in Chapter 2) increases if the athlete returns to sport and sustains a significant trauma prior to complete recovery.

Previous History of Injury

When examining musculoskeletal injuries, clinicians understand that after a ligament or muscle is stretched, it does not typically return to its original position. While there is some debate regarding the cumulative and additive effect of brain injury, researchers believe that there is sufficient evidence to support the thought that the brain does not return to baseline after concussion and it becomes more susceptible to future injuries.[42,55-57] Recent studies have found that athletes with a history of 3 or more concus-sions have a longer recovery and are 4 times more likely to sustain another concussion.[58,59]

While the long-term consequences of concussion are best identified through longitudinal and post-career data, minimal work has been done in the interscholastic and youth setting. There appears to be a deleteri-ous effect of brain function following concussive injury. Individuals with recent concussions performed significantly worse on measures of attention and concentration than youth athletes with no history of concussion.[57,60] Symptom-free youth athletes with a history of 2 or more concussions performed similarly on testing to youth athletes who had just experienced a recent concussion.[57] Collins et al[60] found that athletes with a previous history of concussion and/or learning disability scored significantly lower on neuropsychological tests than those with no previous history of concussion and/or learning disability.

Learning Disabilities

Learning disabilities have been shown to affect executive function.[51,52,61] Executive function includes attention, reasoning, planning, inhibition, set-shifting, interference control, and working memory and is an important aspect of human behavior.[62] Specifically, patients with learning disabilities have also demonstrated consistently worse performance on neuropsychological tests that assess executive functions.[63,64] This trend has been exhibited in traditional pencil-and-paper neuropsychological test scores as well as computerized, short neuropsychological test batteries.

Learning disabilities have been found to affect neuropsychological test scores in all populations with normative values that are typically lower than control group values.[61,65-70] The only existing study[23] specific to concussion found that athletes with a previous history of concussion and/or learning disability scored significantly lower on neuropsychological tests than those with no previous history of concussion and/or learning disability.[60]

Care should be given to those with diagnosed learning disabilities when assessing with neuropsychological tests. Many concussion test batteries include tests of attention and memory. If the subject displays deficits in these areas, these tests should be verified prior to interpretation.

Environmental Influences

Neurocognitive outcomes following injury have been predicted by a patient's family environment, specifically socioeconomic status.[71-73] A study of young children[71] suggests that higher socioeconomic status (SES) is positively correlated with performance on most tests. Although measures of environmental disadvantage predict lower scores on most tests in children with and without severe TBI, these factors may amplify the effects of brain injury on some tests but dampen or obscure effects on other measures.[71,72]

Multiple factors must be considered when evaluating test scores. Neuropsychological test scores among normal, community-living persons can resemble scores of individuals with known neuropsychological impairment due to the effects of comorbidities within the subject.[73-78] Unpublished pilot study data (Hunt TN, Pedroza A, unpublished data, November 2011) provided initial evidence that a lower socioeconomic urban school district has demonstrated cognitive test scores that are 10% lower than published normative data provided by the computerized testing company.

Social Factors

Recovery time may be prolonged when social support is removed and secondary psychological deficits emerge. These deficits could become magnified given the current standard of care that requires cognitive rest while symptomatic. Cognitive rest within the treatment protocol requires patients to disengage from academic and social activities; this has the dire side effect of isolating the athlete from social and physical activities that may be necessary.[79] Given that brain injuries commonly produce depression, adding prescribed isolation may only compound the negative psychological outcomes.[80,81] Sport-related concussion poses additional risks, as the injury itself is associated with a variety of symptoms and the insult to the brain may further hinder appropriate psychological coping and enhance secondary psychological deficits.[78,81] Although most studies examining post-concussion symptoms have focused on somatic complaints,[82,83] athletes can experience psychological distress such as depression, anxiety, frustration, and irritability.[80,83-85]

Psychological and psychiatric symptoms tend to evolve over time, often over a period of weeks to months. Anxiety and affective symptoms may compound and complicate the clinical picture, particularly if the initial symptoms do not dissipate rapidly. Irritability, insomnia, and worry often complicate and amplify pain (eg, headache). Patients with a concussive injury and who have a post-injury recovery course complicated by significant depression report an increased number of symptoms and more severe symptoms than clinically depressed and concussed groups.[79,80]

While some research suggests no difference in depression between concussed and uninjured control groups,[79] increased depression and confusion were evident in concussed athletes compared to their noninjured peers, even though they did not differ from their peers before injury.[46] Providing a management strategy for the psychological response to concussion can aid in rehabilitation, psychosocial development, and efficient recovery.

Effort

Professional athletes have recently admitted to *tanking,* or purposefully performing poorly on baseline tests, in order to return to participation faster. This technique has trickled down with college and high school athletes now beginning to tank baseline tests. Athletes with prior test experience may perform poorly to mask any cognitive changes attributed to a concussive injury. It is well established in the worker's compensation literature[86-90] that an individual's effort may influence neuropsychological scores on baseline performances, thus decreasing neuropsychologists' ability to make adequate clinical interpretations regarding the post-injury assessment following a concussive injury.

It is important for clinicians to discriminate between improvements due to learning, practice effects, poor baseline measures, and improvements due to recovery from mild head injury. In concussion assessment, it is traditionally assumed that maximal effort is given during all test sessions.[34] If a clinician is not aware of a patient's deliberate poor effort, he or she may overlook decreases in neuropsychological scores due to lack of trying.[86] If an athlete does not put forth his or her best effort, baseline scores are not comparable and, therefore, a direct interpretation of post-injury data cannot be made.[34] Hunt et al[91] examined whether maximal effort is given during baseline testing and found that 11% of athletes performed poorly regardless of other comorbidities. Further, poor effort resulted in lower neuropsychological test scores when compared to the students' age-matched normal peers.[91] While few studies have examined effort in the sport-concussion literature, effort may play a large role in decreasing test scores and should be considered a modifying factor.

Summary

- The majority of concussions will recover in a normal fashion (spontaneously over several days).

- Limit the amount of exertion (physical and mental) to allow the brain to heal.

- While evidence supports the use of some medications for specific concussion symptoms, there is no pharmacological treatment approved for concussion in the United States.

- A few pharmacological treatments have provided evidence to specific concussion symptoms such as sleep disturbances, headache, and nausea.

- Recovery may be prolonged by numerous modifying factors including age, improper management, previous history of concussion, learning disabilities, environmental factors, and social factors.

- Proper counseling of expectations following injury should be conducted to ensure that the athlete understands why he or she may be different from another athlete with a concussion.

References

1. Sbordone RJ. A conceptual model of nueropsychologically-based cognitive rehabilitation. In: Williams JM, Long CJ, eds. *The Rehabiliation of Cognitive Disabilities.* New York, NY: Plenum Press; 1996:1-28.

2. Aubry M, Cantu R, Dvorak J, et al. Summary and agreement statement of the First International Conference on Concussion in Sport, Vienna 2001: recommendations for the improvement of safety and health of athletes who may suffer concussive injuries. *Br J Sports Med.* 2002;36(1):6-10.

3. McCrory P, Johnston K, Meeuwisse W, et al. Summary and agreement statement of the 2nd International Conference on Concussion in Sport, Prague 2004. *Br J Sports Med.* 2005;39(4):196-204.

4. Broglio SP, Macciocchi SN, Ferrara MS. Sensitivity of the concussion assessment battery. *Neurosurgery.* 2007;60:1050-1058.

5. Valentine V, Logan K. Cognitive rest in concussion management. *Am Fam Physician.* 2012;85(2):100-101.

6. Majerske CW, Mihalik JP, Ren D, et al. Concussion in sports: postconcussive activity levels, symptoms and neurocognitive performance. *J Athl Train.* 2008;43:265-274.

7. Moser RS, Glatts C, Schatz P. Efficacy of immediate and delayed cognitive and physical rest for treatment of sports-related concussion. *J Pediatr.* 2012;161(5):922-926.

8. Petraglia AL, Maroon JC, Bailes JE. From the field of play to the field of combat: a review of the pharmacological management of concussion. *Neurosurgery.* 2012;70(6):1520-1533.

9. Meehan WP III. Medical therapies for concussion. *Clin Sports Med.* 2011;30(1):115-124.

10. Maiese K, Chong ZZ. Nicotinamide: necessary nutrient emerges as a novel cytoprotectant for the brain. *Trends Pharmacol Sci.* 2003;24(5):228-232.

11. Vagnozzi R, Tavazzi B, Signoretti S, et al. Window of metabolic brain vulnerability to concussions: mitochondrial-related impairment—Part I. *Neurosurgery.* 2007;61(2):379-389.

12. Hoane MR, Akstulewicz SL, Toppen J. Treatment with vitamin B3 improves functional recovery and reduces GFAP expression following traumatic brain injury in the rat. *J Neurotrauma.* 2003;20(11):1189-1199.

13. Tyler GS, McNeely HE, Dick ML. Treatment of post-traumatic headache with amitriptyline. *Headache.* 1980;20:213-216.

14. Label L. Treatment of post-traumatic headaches: maprotiline or amitriptyline? *Neurology.* 1991;41(suppl 1):247.

15. Saran A. Antidepressants not effective in headache associated with minor closed head injury. *Int J Psychiatry Med.* 1988;18:75-83.

16. Tyler GS, McNeely HE, Dick ML. Treatment of post-traumatic headache with amitryptiline. *Headache.* 1980;20:213–216.

17. Jicha GA, Markesbery WR. Omega-3 fatty acids: potential role in the management of early Alzheimer's disease. *Clin Inter Aging.* 2010;5:45-61.

18. Mills JD, Hadley K, Bailes JE. Dietary supplementation with the omega-3 fatty acid docosahexaenoic acid in traumatic brain injury. *Neurosurgery.* 2011;68(2):474-481.

19. Rockswold G, Ford S, Anderson D. Results of a prospective randomized trial for the treatment of severely brain injured patients with hyperbaric oxygen. *Neurosurgery.* 1992;76:929-934.

20. Hargens AR, Schmidt DA, Evans KL, et al. Quantitation of skeletal-muscle necrosis in a model compartment syndrome. *J Bone Joint Surg Am.* 1981;63(4):631-636.

21. Pierce AK. Assisted respiration. *Annu Rev Med.* 1969;20:431-448.

22. Bird AD, Telfer AB. Effect of hyperbaric oxygen on limb circulation. *Lancet.* 1965;1(7381):355-356.

23. Nylander G, Nordstrom H, Eriksson E. Effects of hyperbaric oxygen on oedema formation after a scald burn. *Burns Incl Therm Inj.* 1984;10(3):193-196.

24. Neubauer RA, Gottlieb SF, Pevsner NH. Hyperbaric oxygen for treatment of closed head injury. *South Med J.* 1994;87(9):933-936.

25. Neubauer RA, James P. Cerebral oxygenation and the recoverable brain. *Neurol Res.* 1998;20(suppl 1):S33-S36.

26. Wright JK, Zant E, Groom K, Schlegel RE, Gilliland K. Case report: treatment of mild traumatic brain injury with hyperbaric oxygen. *Undersea Hyperb Med.* 2009;36(6):391-399.

27. Rigg JL, Elovic EP, Greenwald BD. A review of the effectiveness of antioxidant therapy to reduce neuronal damage in acute traumatic brain injury. *J Head Trauma Rehabil.* 2005;20(4):389-391.

28. Hallenbeck J, Jacobs T, Faden A. Combined PGI2, indomethacin and heparin improves neurological recovery after spinal trauma in cats. *J Neurosurg.* 1983;58:749-754.

29. Teasdale G, Bailey I, Bell A, et al. A randomized trial of nimodipine in severe head injury: HIT I. British/Finnish Cooperative Head Injury Trial Group. *J Neurotrauma.* 1991;9(suppl 2):S545-S550.

30. Compton J, Lee T, Jones N. A double blind placebo controlled trial of the calcium entry blocking drug nicardipine in the treatment of vasospasm following severe head injury. *Br J Neurosurg.* 1990;4:9-16.

31. Parker RS. *Concussive Brain Trauma: Neurobehavioral Impairment and Maladaption.* Boca Raton, FL: CRC Press Incorporated; 2001.

32. Obrzut JE, Hynd GW. *Child Neuropsychology.* San Diego, CA: Academic Press Inc; 1986:18-26.

33. Anderson VA, Morse SA, Klug G, et al. Predicting recovery from head injury in young children: a prospective analysis. *J Int Neuropsychol Soc.* 1997;3(6):568-580.

34. Hunt TN. The psychometric properties of concussion assessment tools in high school athletics [dissertation]. Athens, GA: University of Georgia; 2006.

35. Guskiewicz KM, Weaver NL, Padua DA, et al. Epidemiology of concussion in collegiate and high school football players. *Am J Sports Med.* 2000;28(5):643-650.

36. McCrea M, Hammeke T, Olsen G, Leo P, Guskiewicz K. Unreported concussion in high school football players: implications for prevention. *Clin J Sport Med.* 2004;14(1):13-17.

37. Pellman EJ, Lovell MR, Viano DC, Casson IR, Tucker AM. Concussion in professional football: neuropsychological testing—Part 6. *Neurosurgery.* 2004;55(6):1290-1303.

38. Barth J, Alves W, Ryan T, et al. Mild head injury in sports: neuropsychological sequelae and recovery of function. In: Levin H, Eisenber H, Benton A, eds. *Mild Head Injury.* New York, NY: Oxford University Press; 1989:257-275.

39. Lovell MR, Collins MW. Neuropsychological assessment of the college football player. *J Head Trauma Rehabil.* 1998;13:9-26.

40. Donders J, Strom D. Neurobehavioral recovery after pediatric head trauma: injury, pre-injury, and post-injury issues. *J Head Trauma Rehabil.* 2000;15(20):792-803.

41. Lovell MR, Collins MW, Iverson GL, et al. Recovery from mild concussion in high school athletes. *J Neurosurg.* 2003;98(2):296-301.

42. Pellman EJ, Viano DC, Tucker AM, Casson IR, Waeckerle JF. Concussion in professional football: reconstruction of game impacts and injuries. *Neurosurgery.* 2003;53:799-814.

43. Field M, Collins MW, Lovell MR, et al. Does age play a role in recovery from sports-related concussion? A comparison of high school and collegiate athletes. *J Pediatr.* 2003;142(5):546-553.

44. Iverson GL. Outcome from mild traumatic brain injury. *Curr Opin Psychiatry.* 2005;18:301-317.

45. Lovell MR, Collins MW, Iverson GL, et al. Recovery from mild concussion in high school athletes. *Neurosurgery.* 2001;98(2):296-301.

46. Collins MW, Iverson GL, Lovell MR, et al. On-field predictors of neuropsychological and symptom deficit following sports-related concussion. *Clin J Sport Med.* 2003;13(4):222-229.

47. Daniel JC, Olesniewicz MH, Reeves DL, et al. Repeated measures of cognitive processing efficiency in adolescent athletes: implications for monitoring recovery from concussion. *Neuropsychiatry Neuropsychol Behav Neurol.* 1999;12(3):167-169.

48. Covassin T, Elbin RJ, Harris W, Parker T, Kontos A. The role of age and sex in symptoms, neurocognitive performance, and postural stability in athletes after concussion. *Am J Sports Med.* 2012;40(6):1303-1312.

49. McClincy MP, Lovell MR, Pardini J, Collins MW, Spore MK. Recovery from sports concussion in high school and collegiate athletes. *Brain Inj.* 2006;20(1):33-39.

50. Giza CC, Hovda DA. The neurometabolic cascade of concussion. *J Athl Train.* 2001;36(3):228-235.

51. Spreen O, Strauss E. *A Compendium of Neuropsychological Tests: Administration, Norms, and Commentary.* 2nd ed. New York: Oxford University Press; 1998.

52. Dacey RG, Vollmer D, Dikmen SS. Mild head injury. In: Cooper PR, ed. *Head Injury.* 3rd ed. Baltimore, MD: Williams and Wilkins; 1993:159-182.

53. Longhi L, Saatman KE, Fujimoto S, et al. Temporal window of vulnerability to repetitive experimental concussive brain injury. *Neurosurgery.* 2005;56(2):364-374.

54. Greisbach GS, Gomez-Pinilla F, Hovda DA. Time window for voluntary exercise induces increases in hippocampal neuroplasticity molecules after traumatic brain injury in severity dependent. *J Neurotrauma.* 2007;24:1161-1171.

55. Asplund CA, McKeag DB, Olsen CH. Sport-related concussion: factors associated with prolonged return to play. *Clin J Sport Med.* 2004;14(6):339-343.

56. Swaine BR, Tremblay C, Platt RW, Grimard G, Zhang X, Pless BI. Previous head injury is a risk factor for subsequent head injury in children: a longitudinal cohort study. *Pediatrics.* 2007;119(4):749-758.

57. Moser RS, Schatz P. Enduring effects of concussion in youth athletes. *Arch Clin Neuropsychol.* 2002;17(1):91-100.

58. Guskiewicz KM, Marshall SW, Broglio SP, Cantu RC, Kirkendall DT. No evidence of impaired neurocognitive performance in collegiate soccer players. *Am J Sports Med.* 2002;30(2):157-162.

59. McCrea M, Guskiewicz KM, Marshall SW, et al. Acute effects and recovery time following concussion in collegiate football players: the NCAA concussion study. *JAMA.* 2003;290(19):2556-2563.

60. Collins MW, Grindel SH, Lovell MR, et al. Relationship between concussion and neuropsychological performance in college football players. *JAMA*. 1999;282(10):964-970.

61. Jakobson A, Kikas E. Cognitive functioning in children with and without attention-deficit/hyperactivity disorder with and without comorbid learning disabilities. *J Learning Disabil.* 2007;40(3):194-202.

62. Jurado MB, Rosselli M. The elusive nature of executive functions: a review of our current understanding. *Neuropsychol Rev.* 2007;17(3):213-233.

63. Passler MA, Isaac W, Hynd GW. Neuropsychological development of behavior attributed to frontal lobe functioning in children. *Dev Neuropsychol.* 1985;1(4):349-370.

64. Hunt TN, Ferrara MS. Age-related differences in neuropsychological testing among high school athletes. *J Athl Train.* 2009;44(4):405-409.

65. Beers SR, Goldstein G, Katz LJ. Neuropsychological differences between college students with learning disabilities and those with mild head injury. *J Learning Disabil.* 1994;27(5):315-324.

66. Segalowitz SJ, Brown D. Mild head injury as a source of developmental disabilities. *J Learning Disabil.* 1991;24(9):551-559.

67. Seidman LJ, Biederman J, Monuteaux MC, Weber W, Faraone SV. Neuropsychological functioning in nonreferred siblings of children with attention deficit/hyperactivity disorder. *J Abnorm Psychol.* 2000;109(2):252-265.

68. Slomine BS, Salorio CF, Grados MA, Vasa RA, Christensen JR, Gerring JP. Differences in attention, executive functioning, and memory in children with and without ADHD after severe traumatic brain injury. *J Int Neuropsychol Soc.* 2005;11(5):645-653.

69. Anderson VA, Catroppa C, Dudgeon P, et al. Understanding predictors of functional recovery and outcome 30 months following early childhood head injury. *Neuropsychology.* 2006;20(1):42-57.

70. Taylor HG, Yeates KO, Wade SL, et al. Influences on first-year recovery from traumatic brain injury in children. *Neuropsychology.* 1999;13(1):76-89.

71. Kennepohl S, Shore D, Nabors N, et al. African American acculturation and neuropsychological test performance following traumatic brain injury. *J Int Neuropsychol Soc.* 2004;10:566-577.

72. Baxendale S, Heaney D. Socioeconomic status, cognition and hippocampal sclerosis. *Epilepsy Behav.* 2011;20:64-67.

73. Paxson C, Schady N. Cognitive development among young children in Ecuador: the roles of wealth, health and parenting. World Bank Policy Research Paper 3605. Washington, DC: The World Bank Development Research Group; 2005.

74. Greiffenstein MF, Baker WJ. Premorbid clues? Pre-injury scholastic performance and present neuropsychological functioning in late postconcussion syndrome. *Clin Neuropsych.* 2003;17(4):561-573.

75. Rutter M, Chadwick O, Shaffer D. Head injury. In: Rutter M, ed. *Developmental Neuropsychiatry.* New York, NY: Guilford Press; 1983:83-111.

76. Paniak C, Reynolds S, Toller-Lobe G, Melnyk A, Nagy J, Schmidt D. A longitudinal study of the relationship between financial compensation and symptoms after treated mild traumatic brain injury. *J Clin Exp Neuropsych.* 2002;24:187-193.

77. Moore EL, Terryberry-Spohr L, Hope DA. Mild traumatic brain injury and anxiety sequelae: a review of the literature. *Brain Inj.* 2006;20:117-132.

78. Kinsella G, Prior M, Sawyer M, et al. Predictors and indicators of academic outcome in children two years following traumatic brain injury. *J Int Neuropsychol Soc.* 1997;3:608-616.

79. Macleod S. Post concussion syndrome: the attraction of the psychological by the organic. *Med Hypotheses.* 2010;74:1033–1035.

80. Mainwaring L. Restoration of self: a model for the psychological response of athletes to severe knee injuries. *Canadian J Rehabil.* 1999;12:145-156.

81. Taylor HG, Dietrich A, Nuss K, et al. Post-concussive symptoms in children with mild traumatic brain injury. *Neuropsychology.* 2010;24(2):148-159.

82. Mailer BJ, Valovich McLeod TC, Bay RCB. Healthy youth are reliable in reporting symptoms on a graded symptom scale. *J Sport Rehabil.* 2008;16:11-20.

83. Mainwaring LM, Bisschop SM, Green RE, et al. Emotional reaction of varsity athletes to sport-related concussion. *J Sport Exer Psych.* 2004;26:t9-t35.

84. Simon G, Von Korff M, Picinelli M, Fullerton C, Ormel J. An international study on the relation between somatic symptoms and depression. *N Engl J Med.* 1999;341:1329-1355.

85. Lange RT, Iverson GL, Rose A. Depression strongly influences postconcussion symptom reporting following mild traumatic brain injury. *J Head Trauma Rehabil.* 2011:26(2):127-137.

86. Faust D, Hart K, Guilmette T, Arkes H. Neuropsychologists' capacity to detect adolescent malingerers. *Professional Psychology: Research and Practice.* 1988;19(5):508-515.

87. Green P, Iverson GL. Effects of injury severity and cognitive exaggeration on olfactory deficits in head injury compensation claims. *Neurorehabilitation.* 2001;16(4):237-243.

88. Green P, Rohling ML, Lees-Haley PR, Allen LM. Effort has a greater effect on test scores than severe brain injury in compensation claimants. *Brain Inj.* 2001;15(12):1045-1060.

89. Iverson GL, Binder LM. Detecting exaggeration and malingering in neuropsychological assessment. *J Head Trauma Rehab.* 2000;15(2):829-858.

90. Sweet JJ. *Forensic Neuropsychology: Fundamentals and Practice.* Exton, PA: Swets & Zeitlinger; 1999.

91. Hunt TN, Ferrara MS, Miller LS, Macciocchi S. The effect of effort on baseline neuropsychological test scores in high school football athletes. *Arch Clin Neuropsych.* 2007;22(5):615-621.

RETURN TO PARTICIPATION GUIDELINES

Health care professionals strive to develop an ideal protocol for concussion assessment and return to participation decisions to ensure the safety of all participants in athletics. It has been noted that 40.5% of high school athletes return to participation too soon after suffering a concussion.[1] As clinicians, it is imperative to understand and inform all members of the sports medicine team about every aspect of concussion assessment and management.

The majority of injuries will be routine concussions, and such injuries recover spontaneously over several days. In these situations, it is expected that an athlete will proceed rapidly through the stepwise return to participation strategy. The goal of return to participation criteria is to provide the clinician with objective information regarding recovery from injury. Clinicians need to make sure that the brain has had a chance to adequately heal to prevent a secondary, and potentially catastrophic, injury.

When developing return to participation guidelines, there should be input from every stakeholder of the sports medicine team. Hunt and Trombley[2] found that 100% of physicians surveyed about return to participation practices stated that it was the team physician's decision on whether an athlete was ready to return to participation.[3] However, in situations where a physician is not accessible, it is the responsibility of other health care professionals to manage these injuries and make an educated decision regarding return to participtation. To ensure adequate care and return to participation, the sports medicine team should have predetermined guidelines to direct the decision-making process in return to participation. These guidelines should meet the following criteria:

- Be constructed prior to the start of any athletic season.

- Be agreed on by all members of the sports medicine team.

- Be taught to everyone working with athletes (coaches, athletes, parents, and administrators).

Hunt TN.
Cram Session in Evaluation of Sports Concussion:
A Handbook for Students & Clinicians (pp. 93-98).
© 2013 Taylor & Francis Group.

- Include as many objective measures as possible in an effort to eliminate human bias and influence.

Return to participation protocols vary from institution, population, and clinician knowledge. The variation typically depends on the training of the medical staff; the tools available to the medical staff; and the relationship that members of the medical staff have with the athletes, coaches, and administration.

Individual variability associated with symptom report and dysfunction during concussive injuries makes it essential to perform objective testing to ensure the deficits in each domain have returned to normal. It is crucial that no deficits are present when increasing activity to ensure safe return to participation. Therefore, a multifaceted approach is suggested to support return to participation decisions. This should include tests that were utilized during baseline testing (or when baseline testing is not available, utilize tests in as many domains available to the institution such as cognitive, balance, self-reported symptoms, physical examination, and neurological tests).

It has been recommended to perform a stepwise progression that has the following elements[4,5]:

- Increases exertion (mental and physical), slowly

- Is well monitored

- Abides by the professional standard of care and state/federal legislation in the jurisdiction

While individual institutional variations exist, the most commonly followed stepwise protocol is some variation of the progression proposed by the Concussion in Sport group.[4] Many professional organizations and agencies have recommended testing athletes prior to their competitive season for baseline values. The recommended steps are as follows:

- **Step 1:** When a concussion occurs, as diagnosed by certified athletic trainer and/or team physician, clinicians should limit the patient's exertion in normal daily activities. If possible, do not encourage activity, but support cognitive rest.

  ▷ During the first few days following an injury, it is important to emphasize that physical and cognitive rest is required. Activities that require concentration and attention may exacerbate the symptoms and as a result, delay recovery.

▷ The most commonly used clinical protocol, which suggests forego-
ing testing when the athlete is symptomatic, has yet to prove beneficial with high-quality evidence. However, testing may increase
mental exertion and exacerbate symptoms, thus the suggestion to
forego testing.

▷ Give the athlete a self-reported symptom daily checklist until the
athlete is asymptomatic.

- **Step 2:** A 24-hour asymptomatic period prior to testing rather than at the
time of testing is seen.

- **Step 3:** Increase mental exertion.

  ▷ The athlete should be back to regular academic and work activities
  that do not increase physical exertion.

- **Step 4:** Conduct concussion assessment test battery to assess return to
normal function in all domains. When returning to participation, physicians and certified athletic trainers are using a multifaceted approach
that relies heavily on the following:[2,6]

  ▷ Physical examination

  ▷ Cognitive test

  ▷ Balance test

  ▷ Neurological test

  ▷ Other

- **Step 5:** Light aerobic exercise, such as walking or stationary cycling; no
resistance training.

  ▷ An additional consideration in return to participation is that concussed athletes should not only be asymptomatic but also should
  not be taking any pharmacological agents or medications that may
  affect or modify the symptoms of concussion.

  ▷ The goal of this stage is to minimize contact (including ground
  reaction forces from running on pavement) while increasing heart
  rate and metabolic demand.

  ▷ The clinician should observe the athlete during the increase in
  heart rate as well as during cool down.

  ▷ At this point, the athlete should avoid resistance training.
  Resistance training can increase symptoms. When returning to

resistance training, clinicians should pay close attention to proper lifting technique. Ensure the athlete is not holding his or her breath during lifts, as this will increase blood pressure, which may exacerbate symptoms.

- **Step 6:** Sport-specific exercise (eg, skating in hockey, running, or dribbling in soccer) and initiation of resistance training.

  ▷ Clinicians should ensure that proper lifting techniques and proper breathing techniques are being completed during resistance training.

  ▷ At this point, it is still important to avoid contact.

- **Step 7:** Noncontact training drills.

  ▷ Progression of resistance training should be continued at this step.

- **Step 8:** Full contact training after medical clearance.

- **Step 9:** Game play.

Figure 5-1 shows a return to participation concussion stepwise protocol.

The clinician should pay careful attention to the athlete following every step of the progression. It is important to ensure that the athlete is still asymptomatic after exertion.

There has been some debate regarding the presentation of symptoms during the stepwise protocol and the need to go back to the previous step or to a period of rest. Some suggest that the patient should drop back to the previous asymptomatic level and try to progress again after 24 hours. The author suggests erring on the side of caution: if symptoms appear, complete recovery has not occurred and the athlete may have begun the progression too soon. Therefore, patients should go back to the rest period and begin again after symptoms have subsided.

Summary

- Recovery should be examined using a multifaceted assessment before the return to participation progression is started.

- When return to participation is initiated, it should be progressed slowly by first increasing mental exertion followed by physical exertion.

- A stepwise progression should be followed, with clinicians paying close attention to symptom increases.

- Complete recovery should be determined by the return to normal/baseline on multifaceted concussion assessment tools.

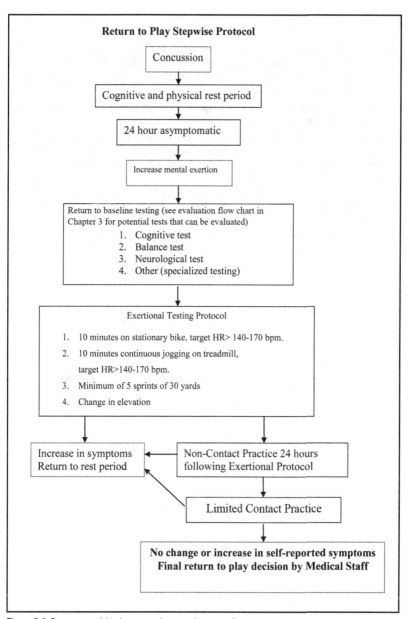

Figure 5-1. Return to participation concussion stepwise protocol.

References

1. Yard EE, Comstock RD. Compliance with return to play guidelines following concussion in US high school athletes, 2005-2008. *Brain Inj.* 2009;23(11):888-898.

2. Mailer BJ, Valovich McLeod TC, Bay RCB. Healthy youth are reliable in reporting symptoms on a graded symptom scale. *J Sport Rehabil.* 2008;16:11-20.

3. Hunt TN, Trombley A. Physician management of sport-related concussion at the collegiate level. *Athl Train Sports Health Care.* 2010;2:227-234.

4. Aubry M, Cantu R, Dvorak J, et al. Summary and agreement statement of the First International Conference on Concussion in Sport, Vienna 2001: recommendations for the improvement of safety and health of athletes who may suffer concussive injuries. *Br J Sports Med.* 2002;36(1):6-10.

5. Guskiewicz KM, Bruce SL, Cantu R, et al. National Athletic Trainers' Association position statement: management of sport-related concussion. *J Athl Train.* 2004;39(3):280-297.

6. Piland SG, Motl RW, Guskiewicz KM, McCrea M, Ferrara MS. Structural validity of a self-report concussion related symptom scale. *Med Sci Sports Exer.* 2006;38:27–32.

RETURN TO SCHOOL/WORK ACCOMMODATIONS

It is crucial for the well-being of all athletes to ensure that the sports medicine team is all-inclusive. Discussions continue to focus on creating and working in a multidisciplinary team for assessment, management, and return to participation; however, it is most important when returning an athlete to academics and work. Clinicians have utilized psychologists, counselors, and administrators and have provided additional access to support structures that are not always available to health care professionals. As the support of a concussed athlete does not stop when he or she leaves the athletic venue, team members must consider how the injury affects every aspect of the athlete's life. This includes social support, academic support, and employment support. This chapter will focus on support structures that clinicians can use when helping patients transition back to school or work.

As health care providers, clinicians traditionally work within systems as a link in communication to provide the most support for the patient. When discussing transitioning back into academics, the relationship between health care providers and the school district can modify the trust, support, and eventually the willingness to cooperate with any accommodations the student may need. When returning to school, this relationship must include the athlete's teachers, administrators, counselors, nurses, and psychologists.

It is imperative to work with the school district and employer to establish a return to work and/or school plan that incorporates feedback from all parties involved. Communication is enhanced when the school and work administration can provide equal input into the return to participation and/or academics protocol. Every stake holder should have some buy in for developing a reintegration plan that works for everyone. A cooperative and collaborative approach to identify and implement appropriate accommodations for those recovering from concussions is crucial to a successful recovery. Compliance with return to work and school guidelines will be improved if the administrators are aware of the limitations and work to provide appropriate accommodations so health care is continuous and complete.

Hunt TN.
Cram Session in Evaluation of Sports Concussion:
A Handbook for Students & Clinicians (pp. 99-105).
© 2013 Taylor & Francis Group.

When working with a patient who has a concussion, the clinician can find additional support from the Americans with Disabilities Act (ADA).[1] The ADA was passed in 1990 and borrows from the 504 definition of a disabled person (ie, an individual who has a physical or mental impairment, a record of impairment, or is regarded as having impairment).[1] The ADA applied those standards to most private-sector businesses in an effort to eliminate barriers to disabled access in buildings, transportation, and communication. The ADA has been revised and supplemented for educational institutions and the incorporation of the Individuals with Disabilities Education Act (IDEA).[1]

Within the IDEA, written accommodations are identified through an individual education program (IEP).[1] An IEP is designed to meet the unique educational needs of one child, who may have a disability as defined by federal regulations. The IEP is intended to help children reach educational goals more easily than they otherwise would. Most commonly, IEPs are utilized for student-athletes who sustain a concussion and do not recover in a timely fashion, and as a result of the injury have long-lasting and/or severe cognitive deficits that impact academics. This is commonly seen in patients who sustain a concussion and progress to post-concussion syndrome with prolonged cognitive and psychosocial deficits.

Because the symptoms and effects of concussions are transient in nature, long-term accommodations are typically not warranted. Because of this, an IEP is not always the best option. Schools can instead chose to initiate a 504 plan, which is a temporary adjustment/accommodation period for academics. It is similar to but often shorter than an IEP. Clinicians should not rush into implementing a written 504 plan if the school and teachers are making appropriate accommodations, but when there is a lack of support, a written plan may be the most appropriate action.

Many types of accommodations can be provided by health care professionals but are typically associated with the presentation of symptoms. The initial accommodations should start during a clinical visit when the clinician should educate the student-athlete and guardians to avoid performing activities that exacerbate symptoms. This should include the use of technology such as watching television, instant messaging, texting, computer time, and/or playing video games. If possible, student-athletes should only perform activities when they are symptom-free. Additional education should include management strategies for returning to school. The clinician may recommend excused absences from school or excused from specific classes during the acute phase of the injury. During this phase, the student should be encouraged to get as much sleep and rest as possible. This may include

September 2, 2004

RE: Little Jane Smith

To Whom It May Concern:

This patient has suffered a concussion approximately 2 weeks ago. She was examined at the OSU Sports Concussion on August18, 2004. She continues to be symptomatic and is being withheld from athletic activity until her symptoms resolve. Her post-concussion symptoms will also potentially interfere with her academic performance. Until her symptoms resolve she should be allowed to use a tape recorder for her classes. She should be allowed to postpone examinations until her symptoms resolve. If examinations cannot be postponed, she should be given additional time for examinations, and should be allowed to take a break during examination sessions. She should work with another student to share notes, and should be allowed to rest during his study hall periods. If possible her classes should be re-organized to allow her to have a break between strongly academic subjects. If this is not possible, she should be allowed to have a break between classes (such as coming 10-15 minutes late to class) or leaving the classroom for a brief break during these classes. She should not take physical education classes for the remainder of this academic year. These accommodations should continue until her symptoms resolve and she is released for return to athletic activity.

Please feel free to contact me if you have any questions.

Sincerely,

Joe Schmoe, MD
Sports Medicine Center
Sports Concussion Program

Figure 6-1. Sample school accommodation letter.

sleeping for longer hours (eg, going to bed early and sleeping in), while still performing some activities of daily living.

The goal is to enhance student transition and support back into academia. As symptoms decrease, clinicians may suggest only attending school if headaches and symptoms are absent or at a low-level, and the athlete has the ability to concentrate without increasing symptoms. Figure 6-1 provides a sample letter that may be provided to the athlete's school. The initial return to school may occur in quarter- or half-days. The student may need to alternate morning and afternoon attendance to cover all classes and not miss subjects entirely while trying to avoid going to all of his or her most challenging classes at one time. Lastly, the athlete should be excused from physical activity, such as gym classes and sports.

Once the athlete is cleared to return to school, the initial step is to work with his or her teachers to provide appropriate accommodations for the injured athlete. The goal is to get the most out of the school day without worsening symptoms. The following concepts can be utilized to aid recovery and include, but are not limited to, the following:

- Optimize learning without creating quick fatigue
  - Reading and math have been shown to cause symptoms
  - Temporary tutor or assistance for more difficult courses
  - Do not take notes in class
    * Use of a note taker or scribe
    * Use of a reader for assignment and testing
  - Listening to lectures only
  - Limit computer time
- Watch for over-stimulation
  - Avoid loud hallways, cafeterias, and recess areas
  - Leave class prior to the bell to avoid crowded hallways and over-stimulation during the initial recovery period
  - Decrease sound and light exposure
    * Avoid music classes, woodshop class, and the cafeteria. The student-athlete may also benefit from wearing earplugs or hats/sunglasses to decrease light and sound exposure
  - Accommodation for classroom seating
    * Move the student closer to the chalk board
  - Allow for rest in nurse's office, as needed
  - Provide time to go to study hall or a quiet place to get cognitive rest during the day. This can give the athlete relief if symptoms increase throughout the course of the day
- Provide support for assignments or examinations
  - Postpone homework, tests, and papers
  - Ask for an extension of assignment deadlines

▷ Short bursts of homework can be attempted. Work for 20-minute intervals if possible

▷ Postpone or stagger tests until full cognitive recovery has occurred (especially standardized testing)

▷ Excuse from specific tests and assignments that are less crucial for grading

▷ Provide a smaller, quieter room for assignments or examinations to reduce stimulation and distraction

▷ Extended test time

When returning patients to work, the clinician should start with counseling in the office to evaluate signs and symptom exacerbation from either excessive mental or physical exertion. Several studies examining return to work for various severities of patients with brain injury found rates of 12% to 66% of patients returned to full premorbid level of employment.[2,3] An additional 30% returned to modified work.[2,3] Special attention should be given to patients with complicated family lives, unstable home environments, and additional comorbidities such as psychiatric conditions.[4] Additional consideration should be explained when returning to work requires physical exertion.

Clinicians should be aware of administrative requirements for accommodations in the workplace. Communication with the patient should include whether it is appropriate for the patient to return to work temporarily or if additional accommodations can be made. There are several federal and state-related policies that may be utilized for recovery from injury.

In most situations, employees can typically utilize sick leave to cover time away from work while recovering from concussion. If sick leave is not available, short-term disability may be available to supplement pay when the patient is not working full-time. Clinicians should communicate with the patient to determine if short-term disability is available and what necessary documentation the clinician may need to provide. If the injury persists, the patient may be able to utilize the Family Medical Leave Act to protect his or her job while injured. (More information regarding the Family Medical Leave Act can be found at www.dol.gov/whd/fmla). While the law was enacted to protect the employee, there is a requirement that the employee be employed by the organization for at least 1 year before attempting to apply. If the injury occurred as a function of work, additional paperwork may be necessary to certify worker's compensation plans.

If the patient is unable to take time off of work, even with appropriate written documentation from a clinician, some work accommodations may aid in recovery. Some accommodations that can be suggested include but are not limited to the following:

- Working in a quiet environment where the patient can dim the light or muffle the sounds

- Alternative work schedule that enables the patient to obtain more sleep

  ▹ Come in late and leave early if necessary

- Being able to take breaks to avoid excessive stress after performing tasks throughout the day

- In positions that require standing during the day, provide a chair to decrease physical exertion

- Decrease time working on the computer

  ▹ Provide a break during the day

  ▹ Place head down on desk for a short period of time to decrease mental exertion

Summary

- Return to school and work should be completed in a stepwise progression dictated by the presence and recurrence of symptoms.

- Federal- and state-approved accommodations guided by the ADA such as the Family Medical Leave Act, IEPs, and 504 plans are available and at times appropriate for patients recovering from a concussive injury.

- Clinicians should know the available accommodations and support for patients following concussion.

- Communication with all parties involved is key when counseling patients regarding return to school and/or work.

References

1. Walk EE, Ahn HC, Lampkin PM, Nabizadeh SA, Edlich RF. Americans with disabilities act. *J Burn Care Res.* 1993;14(1):91-98.

2. Ruffolo C, Freidland J, Dawson D, Colantonio A, Lindsay P. Mild TBI from motor vehicle accidents: factors associated with return to work. *Arch Phys Med Rehabil.* 1999;80:392-398.

3. Rao N, Rosenthal M, Cronin-Stubbs D, Lambert R, Barnes P, Swanson B. Return to work after rehabilitation following traumatic brain injury. *Brain Inj.* 1990;4(1):49-56.

4. Shames J, Treger I, Haim R, Giaquinto S. Return to work following traumatic brain injury: trends and challenges. *Disabil Rehabil.* 2007;29(17):1387-1395.

7

LEGAL PRECEDENT AND CASES

Recent legislation that requires medical care for all athletes who have sustained concussion necessitates a thorough understanding of short-term and long-term effects, recovery curves, and assessment techniques for concussive injuries. However, the legal ramifications of concussive injuries have hit the media forefront with cases against Division 1 programs for the handling of high-profile athletes.

Federal and State Legislation

Despite recent media coverage to the contrary, there has always been a legal consequence to health care providers for providing poor care to athletes. When treating a patient with a head injury, a physician "has a legal duty to have and use the knowledge, skill, and care ordinarily possessed and used by members of his or her particular specialty in good standing, considering the state of medical science at the time such care is rendered."[1] Recently, it has been suggested that courts in the United States will likely find the National Athletic Trainers' Association (NATA) guidelines the standard of care for management and care of concussed athletes.[1] An athletic trainer who fails to meet the NATA guidelines when evaluating an athlete and who fails to refer the injured athlete to a physician may be liable for negligence as a consequence of such failures. Additional guidelines for other health care professionals will be dictated by their practice acts, standard of care, and appropriate legislation. While federal legislation was developed and pushed for in 2010 (Protecting Student-Athletes from Concussion Act of 2010, HR 6172, 111th Leg), revised, and reintroduced in 2011 (Protecting Student-Athletes from Concussion Act of 2011, HR 469, 112th Leg), it has not been passed at the time of this writing (status: referred to the Subcommittee on Early Childhood, Elementary, and Secondary Education).

Head injury legislation across multiple states has led to changes in the medical management of these injuries. In 2009, Washington (Zackery Lystedt Law, HR 1824, 61st Leg, [WA 2009]) and Oregon (Safety of School Sports—Concussions, ORS 336.485 [2011; Max's Law OAR 581-022-0421]) were the first 2 states to pass concussion laws relating to youth athletics. To

Hunt TN.
Cram Session in Evaluation of Sports Concussion:
A Handbook for Students & Clinicians (pp. 107-118).
© 2013 Taylor & Francis Group.

date, 43 states have passed legislation that requires some form of medical clearance, educational intervention, and management plan implementation. While individual state legislation may differ in exact language, it generally provides guidance for the following:

- If a concussion is diagnosed, the athlete must immediately be removed from play and cannot return to participation the same day.

- Outlines who can provide sideline assessment and return to participation clearance.

- Outlines the minimum education requirement of coaches, parents, athletes, and administrators.

- Stipulates the requirement for developing and implementing a concussion management plan.

While some state legislation is stricter and more concise than others, the clinician should pay close attention to the individual differences afforded by his or her state. All legislation that has currently been passed or introduced is directed specifically toward youth athletics. Currently, clinicians' practice management plans are being guided by current state legislation. In states without legislation, the clinician should refer to the National Federation of State High School Associations (NFHS), professional, and/or local standards. For other populations, several agencies have mandated guidelines for the safety and well-being of athletes when suffering from concussion and returning to participation.

National Federation of State High School Associations

The NFHS Sports Medicine Advisory Board has issued rule changes that affect all NFHS interscholastic athletes as of 2009.[2] Effective for the 2010 to 2011 rulebooks, concussion guidelines recommend the following:

- Any athletic official is permitted to remove a player from the field of play if the athlete demonstrates any signs of concussion.

- Once removed from play, the athlete cannot be returned to play the same day.

- Athletes must be evaluated and eventually cleared by a trained medical professional in order to return to participation.

- Inform the athlete's parents or guardians about the possible concussion and provide education on concussion.

- After clearance is obtained for the athlete to return to participation, a stepwise progression based upon the occurrence of symptoms.

The NFHS has followed the rules and guidelines that were introduced in the Zackery Lystedt legislation in combination with recommendations from the Sports Medicine Advisory Board. While the NFHS is the highest form of a legislative body for interscholastic athletics, the NFHS does not have authority over all institutions. The NFHS can make recommendations, but it is each state's interscholastic association that sets the state policy. Currently, many state interscholastic associations are following the guidelines set forth by the NFHS, though there are some exceptions. The practicing clinician should obtain the most current and relevant information associated with his or her state, local, and institutional recommendations to provide the best quality health care to athletes following concussion.

National Collegiate Athletic Association Recommendations

Increased media attention regarding concussion occurrence and management in high schools and professional sports led to the National Collegiate Athletic Association (NCAA) revising the sports medicine handbook and policies to include updated guidelines on concussion management. While the focus on legislation has been on high school athletes and new rule mandates for the National Football League (NFL)-covered professional athletes, the collegiate ranks were otherwise neglected. Therefore, in 2009, the NCAA mandated that all NCAA participating colleges and universities have a concussion management program in place by the 2010-2011 academic year.[3] NCAA provisions stipulate the following:

- Any student-athlete who exhibits signs, symptoms, or behaviors consistent with a concussion shall be removed from practice or competition and evaluated by an athletics health care provider with experience in the evaluation and treatment as specified by the management plan.

- Student-athletes diagnosed with a concussion shall not return to participation for the remainder of that day.

- Medical clearance shall be determined by the team physician or his or her designee according to the concussion.

- Student-athletes must sign a statement in which they accept the responsibility for reporting their injuries and illnesses to the institutional medical staff, including signs and symptoms of concussions.

- During the review and signing process, student-athletes should be presented with educational material on concussions.

While each state, profession, institution, and school system has begun to acknowledge the importance of appropriate concussion assessment, management, and administration, some individual differences remain. For example, the younger the athlete at the time of injury, the more conservative the management and return to participation decisions. Collegiate athletes must acknowledge responsibility for reporting symptoms and obtaining proper education regarding concussion. While clinicians and researchers are making progress in education, assessment, and management, it is ultimately clinicians and administrators who will establish uniform national concussion standards for all aspects of athletics.

This chapter provides a broad description of the legislation currently in place for concussions in athletics. Specific adaptations of the legislation are dependent on the state, high school association, institution, and professional associations involved with providing care to athletes with concussion. Therefore, it is the clinicians' responsibility to be aware of state and institutional differences and seek information regarding the numerous regulatory layers that go beyond the scope of this book.

Developing a Concussion Management Plan

One major piece of all concussion legislation and management strategies is to develop a concussion management plan. The long-term effects of concussion pose a much greater risk for athletes than other medical conditions in the past, such as diabetes and high blood pressure. Due to the limited knowledge and outcomes for athletes following concussion, clinicians should plan for any eventuality. Clinicians are encouraged to consider concussion management plans equitable to emergency action plans for head injuries. Figure 7-1 is a blank concussion management protocol. Each concussion management plan may be as individual as the institution administration. Clinicians assessing and managing concussive injuries should create a plan that works for the individual athletic population, budget, time constraints, and personnel. However, a basic review to develop a concussion plan is provided in the following sections.

Step 1: Review the Literature Regarding the Population

In this initial step, focus should be placed on the individual needs of the institution. The concussion management team should examine the availability of assessment tools, examine the assessment ability/knowledge of the team, define the concussion management team members (if not already completed), and review examples of concussion management plans from equitable institutions.

Step 2: Draft and Adopt Procedures

A policy on which all members of the sports medicine team can agree should be drafted and adopted. Considered the expert and leader, the team physician should drive the development of this management plan with input from all other members of the concussion management team. Concussion management plans should be as all encompassing as possible. However, all plans should include at least the following:

- A provision stating that if an athlete shows symptoms consistent with a concussion, the athlete shall be removed from practice or competition and evaluated by an athletic health care provider with experience in the evaluation and management of concussive injuries.

- An athlete diagnosed with a concussion shall be withheld from the competition or practice and not return to participation for the remainder of that day.

- Plan for serial monitoring of the athlete for deterioration. This plan should include the type of testing, stipulate who will perform the testing, and how often the testing will occur.

- Stipulate that the decision to return to participation must be made by medical personnel or administration, not coaches.

- Create and foster a "from the top, down" approach to the athlete's safety.

Step 3: Implementation

- Training of all members of the sport management team and athletic support personnel.

- Compose and collect signed waivers (if applicable).

- Provide continuing education and training for the concussion management team and athletic support personnel.

Step 4: Review and Update Evaluation Procedures

- Perform quarterly or yearly analysis to evaluate procedures, update standards, update assessment tools, and plan for the future.

- Analyze how athletic injuries are being handled and if standard of care is accurate/appropriate.

- Identify breakdowns and implement revised procedures if needed.

XYZ Institution

The following document is a team physician driven, concussion policy and management plan that specifically outlines the role of the XYZ sports medicine health care providers. This document has been created and shared with all sports medicine team members and will be the standard policy for all athletes within XYZ institution. All health care professionals within this document agree to practice within the standards as established for their professional practice.

CONCUSSION POLICY

I. Your definition of concussion
>   a. This will have to be an agreed upon definition for all sports medicine staff. A common definition has been the CIS group definition provided below.
>
> Concussion has been defined as "a complex pathophysiological process affecting the brain, induced by traumatic biomechanical forces."[1] This consensus from the 1st international conference for concussion suggested five conditions for concussion.
>>   1. Concussion may be caused either by a direct blow to the head, face, neck or elsewhere on the body with an "impulsive" or rotational force transmitted to the head.
>>   2. Concussion typically results in the rapid onset of short-lived impairment of neurological function that resolves spontaneously.
>>   3. Concussion may result in neuropathological changes, but the acute clinical symptoms rarely reflect a functional disturbance rather than structural injury.
>>   4. Concussion results in a graded set of clinical syndromes that may or may not involve loss of consciousness, resolution of the clinical and cognitive symptoms typically follows a sequential course.
>>>   i. Concussion is typically associated with grossly normal structural neuroimaging studies.
>>>>   a. Who will be tested
>>>>   b. How will they be tested
>>>>   II. Education
>>>>   a. Who will educate
>>>>   b. How often
>>>>   c. When
>>>>   d. What materials will you use to educate:
>>>>>   1. Athletic Trainers
>>>>>   2. Coaches
>>>>>   3. Athletic Directors/Administrators

III. Management Plan
>   a. Baseline Testing
>>   1. When
>>   2. Who
>>   3. How
>>   4. What Tools

Figure 7-1. Concussion management plan.

IV. Time of Injury/Post-Injury
- a. Who will diagnose injury?
- b. How will sports medicine team diagnose injury?
- c. Sideline evaluation
  - 1. When will it occur?
  - 2. How will perform
  - 3. What tools will you utilize?
    - a. Physical Examination
    - b. Neurological Exam
    - c. Cognitive Exam
    - d. Postural Exam
  - 4. Transportation to ER rules
- d. Communication
  - 1. Who will disclose information and to whom
    - a. Athletes
    - b. Parents
    - c. Administration
    - d. Academic support
  - 2. Chain of command
- e. Removal of athlete from activity

V. Post-Injury
- a. Follow-up with whom?
- b. Testing paradigm (when)
- c. Medical clearance
- d. Return to participation progressions
  - 1. Typical progression
  - 2. Who can make changes to progression
  - 3. Rules of progression
  - 4. Visual aid of the progression

VI. Forms
- a. Demographic information sheet
- b. Self-report symptom sheet
- c. Head Injury Take home sheet
- d. Test forms
- e. Documentation

REFERENCE

1.   Aubry M, Cantu R, Dvorak J, et al. Summary and agreement statement of the first International Conference on Concussion in Sport. Vienna, 2001: recommendations for the improvement of safety and health of athletes who may suffer concussive injuries. *Br J Sports Med*. 2002;36(1)6-10.

Figure 7-1 (continued). Concussion management plan.

There are very few organizations that have developed comprehensive concussion programs. One such program is the Reduce, Educate, Accommodate, and Pace (REAP) program.[4] This program was developed by the Rocky Mountain Youth Sports Medicine Institute in Colorado with funding from the Colorado Traumatic Brain Injury Trust Fund. REAP is a community-based concussion management program that has been endorsed by the Colorado High School Activities Association and the Brain Injury Alliance of Colorado.

REAP incorporates medical personnel, academic staff, and the athlete's family as entities to consult in order to enhance communication throughout the process of concussion recovery in adolescent athletes. Developed in 2009, REAP was created with an educational grant to provide instruction to the emergency department and several schools in one school district. After a successful pilot, the program has expanded to include additional school districts and the medical communities that serve them. Additional information for this program can be found at www.cokidswithbraininjury.com/mild-tbi-concussion-info.

Since its inception, several presentations regarding the REAP program have been made and other school districts are hoping to implement a similar multidisciplinary approach to recovery in adolescents. However, funding for a full-time REAP program employee to manage all cases of sport-related concussion and organize care may not be feasible for all school systems and districts. School systems with limited funding will be asked to fulfill the daunting task of providing the same level of care with limited funds. Therefore, an alternative plan that involves a multidisciplinary taskforce already associated with the health care of the student-athlete is provided in Figure 7-2.

The importance of community-based programs must be supported and endorsed by all parties involved. Obtaining feedback from stakeholders in the return to school and participation protocol is an essential part of developing and implementing these programs. Utilization of the resources already available in the school district, such as the school counselors, school psychologists, school nurses, athletic trainers, and physicians will provide the student-athlete with support and appropriate management that will help the athlete return to school and participation safely.

The concussion management protocol is a fluid document that will continue to evolve as technology, staffing, budget, philosophies, and available research changes. Clinicians should remain up-to-date with the latest information to ensure the safest environment possible. As legislation is implemented, the management protocol should be revised to hold all members of

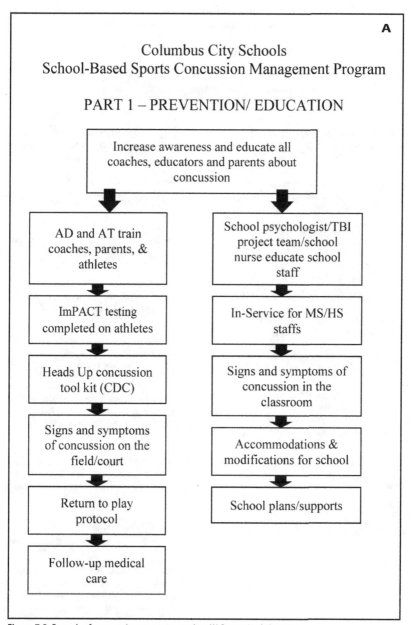

Figure 7-2. Example of a concussion management plan. (A) Prevention/education.

Columbus City Schools
School-Based Sports Concussion Management Program

B

PART 2 – CONCUSSION MANAGEMENT

Student athlete sustains concussion or is suspected of sustaining a concussion during play

Student is immediately removed from play by coach and/or AT	AT notifies School Psych via email/ phone call
Parent signs Release of Information for medical follow-up/ records	School Psych sends home CCS TBI Project brochure on concussion and calls family
Student is given Post-Concussion Symptom Scale to complete daily	School Psych contacts School Contact Person (SCP), principal, teachers and other necessary school personnel
AT notifies principal, coach, & family of concussion	School Psych sends teachers Post-Concussion Symptom Scale to complete for first 2 to 3 weeks post concussion
AT starts file on student: ROI, date and detail of injury, notes of immediate care. Post-Concussion Symptom Sheets, medical advice, etc…	School Psych sends teachers accommodation plan to implement immediately once student returns to school
Log kept of all phone/ face to face conversations: date, with whom, content of, information sheets distributed, etc…	Teachers observe and document what symptoms they observe and return forms to Sch. Psych by Friday of each week
AT checks in daily with student regarding symptoms	SCP checks in daily/ weekly with student regarding symptoms, work load, school performance
AT follows up with doctor on return to play and other recommendations	SCP checks with teachers weekly regarding accommodation plan
	School Psych calls family and consults with AT on symptoms & recovery – if asymptomatic, reduce accommodations slowly until none are needed
	If student is still symptomatic after 3 weeks, school schedules IAT meeting. If symptomatic after 45 days, consider 504 Plan or referral for suspected disability (TBI)

Figure 7-2 (continued). Example of a concussion management plan. (B) Concussion management.

the concussion management team accountable to the federal, state, professional, and institutional standards that had been agreed upon. When all is said and done, clear documentation, expectations, and education will ensure the safety and well-being of every athlete under the clinician's care.

Summary

- Many states across the nation have passed head injury legislation for youth athletics.

- While each state's legislation may have slightly different language, consistent themes for legislation include the following:

  ▷ Education for those involved with athletics.

  ▷ Identification of personnel that can assess, deem recovered, and allow return to participation.

  ▷ Development and institution of a management plan.

- Currently, the legislation only applies to scholastic athletes and younger participants. The NCAA has provided written recommendations for collegiate athletes.

- The clinician's professional organization standards must be met to ensure the team is operating within the scope of practice. Overall, the governing bodies responsible for concussion management include the following:

  ▷ School-aged athletes and younger: State legislation (if available) or the NFHS

  ▷ College-aged athletes: NCAA guidelines

  ▷ Professional athletes: Clinicians should look toward their professional organization's mandates

- Ensure proper documentation of head injuries and that the institution has a concussion management protocol agreed on by the members of the sports medicine team.

References

1. Mitten MJ. 2001 legal issues affecting medical clearance to resume play after mild brain injury. *Clin J Sport Med.* 2001;11:199–202.

2. National Federation of State High Schools Association: Sports Medicine Advisory Committee. *Suggested Guidelines for Management of Concussion in Sports.* Available at: http://www.nfhs.org/content.aspx?id=5786. Revised January 2011. Accessed March 26, 2012.

3. National Collegiate Athletic Association. Concussion. In: *Sports Medicine Handbook.* 22nd ed. Available at: http://www.ncaapublications.com/productdownloads/MD11.pdf. 2011:53-58. Accessed March 26, 2012.

4. Rocky Mountain Youth Sports Medicine Institute Center for Concussion. REAP: The Benefits of Good Concussion Management. Available at: http://www.ochs.orecity.k12. or.us/sites/ochs.orecity.k12.or.us/files/2011-2012-pages/REAP.pdf

8

PREVENTION

Fear of injury and of the long-term consequences of concussion has become the biggest gift to equipment marketing companies. Many companies have jumped on the bandwagon telling parents, administrators, and the general public that their equipment will prevent concussions. Unfortunately, injuries are inherent in sports and there is limited evidence to support the claim that concussions can be prevented. This chapter will briefly discuss the major theories around protective equipment and the evidence for use in concussion management.

Utilization of Headgear and Helmets

The amount of protective equipment on the market for various sports has increased. This includes soccer headgear, girl's lacrosse headgear/helmets, and helmets for pole vaulting.[1-4] However, very limited evidence is available to support claims of a protective effect. Protective headgear has greatly decreased the number and severity of brain injuries in sports, therefore mandating their use,[1,2] but the best tool or protocol has not been elucidated.

Research is ongoing in sports that require headgear. Helmet use appears to reduce head injury risk in skiing, snowboarding, and bicycling,[2,3] but the effect on concussion risk is inconclusive.[4] Evidence supports that the newer helmet models reduce linear acceleration (Gs) and rotational forces compared to not wearing a helmet.[5] This finding may reduce the incidence of diffuse axonal injury but is not conclusive for concussions.[5]

Recent media attention has influenced the use of preventative equipment to avoid the long-term ramifications of head injuries in sports. There are strong correlations to experience level, where the more experienced the player is, the more likely it is that he or she will use headgear.[6,7] Further, evidence is available that supports rugby players who reported always wearing protective headgear during games were at a reduced incident rate of sustaining a concussion.[8,9] However, more recent team evidence examining headgear usage and injury risk reduction was inclusive.[9,10]

Hunt TN.
Cram Session in Evaluation of Sports Concussion:
A Handbook for Students & Clinicians (pp. 119-126).
© 2013 Taylor & Francis Group.

Public opinion suggests wearing any and all protective equipment. However, there are some players who are reluctant to wear headgear due to the stigmas associated with wearing headgear in sports that do not require protective headgear. Taking precautions with head injuries is sometimes seen as not being "tough,"[10,11] leading many players to be concerned about the stigma of using protective equipment. Anecdotally, coaches worry about recklessness.[10] Coaches fear that wearing protective equipment might give athletes a false sense of security or that athletes would use the headgear as a weapon or lead head-first.

Mouth Guards

Mouth guards are thought to provide some preventative effect for concussion by reducing force transmission to the brain via absorption and neck musculature stabilization.[11-15] It is suggested that the posterior thickness of the mouth guard is what prevents the forces to be delivered to the mandible and brain. Unfortunately, the studies[16,17] commonly cited as evidence for mouth guard usage to reduce concussive injuries are case studies and cross-sectional survey research, which are low-level evidence for such a claim.[18-21] Little evidence supports the use of mouth guards or face shields to reduce concussion risk.[15,20,21]

There appears to be limited evidence to support the theory that mouth guards decrease the risk and/or severity of concussions. However, there is evidence that supports the reduction of morbidity and expense resulting from dental injuries.[21] Additionally, there are significant differences between the types of mouth guards and the ability to talk and breathe.[20] Athletes who are more likely to play roles in communication typically prefer custom fit mouth guards, which allow for easier communication. Recommendations for using a mouth guard for dental protection exist[22]; however, conclusive evidence cannot support the use of mouth guards in reducing the incidence of concussion.

Rule Changes

Administrators are constantly trying to identify ways to make athletics safer for those participating. During the 1976 season, the National Collegiate Athletic Association (NCAA) and the National Federation of State High School Associations (NFHS) adopted rules outlawing contact with opposing players using the top of the head (spearing)—a rule change that drastically reduced the number of cervical injuries in athletes.[23,24] Because most injuries occur while tackling or being tackled, the next logical step in research will be to evaluate tackling techniques, educate coaches, and implement improved tackling techniques with players.[25,26]

Recently, ice hockey has changed the rule to require all players to wear a full face mask to protect the head and neck during play. Evidence suggests that full facial protection in ice hockey may reduce concussion severity, as measured by time lost from competition.[27,28] In 2012, the National Football League (NFL) changed the starting position of kickoff because a significant amount of injuries were occurring during this phase of the game. Rule changes will continue to evolve in order to create a safer environment for athletes.

Education

The Zurich consensus and other agency position statements on concussion recognized that education of the athlete, referee, administrators, parents, coaches, and health care providers is a mainstay of progress in this field.[29-32] Moreover, agencies with position statements support that education may be the cornerstone to prevention. While the initial concussion cannot be prevented, education may encourage an athlete to report a concussion to prevent secondary deficits related to delayed recovery or catastrophic consequences from secondary traumas.

Education has been the focus of treatment management plans in order to prevent and decrease the potential adverse outcomes of concussion. If the clinician does not know proper management techniques, he or she could provide inappropriate instructions for athletes. In a study conducted by Powell et al,[33] 56% of concussions identified by the Centers for Disease Control and Prevention (CDC) criteria for concussion were missed in emergency departments. On release from the emergency department, more than 69.7% of youth athletes hospitalized for concussion were given improper follow-up instructions.[34]

Concussive legislation is being passed across the nation requiring medical clearance for concussed athletes to return to participation. The surge of athletes with concussions will require clinicians competent in concussion assessment and management to comply with legislation. However, the education available to clinicians must become more readily available and comprehensive in order to meet the needs of the athletes.

Unlike the clinician, where education is required for clinical practice, the athlete engaging in sports does not follow the same requirement. McCrea et al,[35] found that 53% of athletes do not report concussions. There are a host of reasons why athletes claim they did not report the injury. However, current literature provides evidence that the major reason was that the athlete did not recognize the symptoms as a concussion.[35] Valovich et al[36] found that 25% of athletes reported a history of "getting dinged" or "having their bell rung," but only 8% reported a previous history of concussion. Kaut[37] found 56% of all athletes studied, including soccer players and female athletes, reported no knowledge of the possible consequences following a head injury. This lack of concussion knowledge for athletes affects reporting rates, prompt treatment, and management, which can ultimately influence recovery.

Educating athletes can provide information regarding the need to report the injury and symptoms. Bramley et al[38] found that high school soccer players with knowledge of concussion were more likely to report a concussion to a coach or athletic trainer compared to those athletes with no concussion education. Enabling athletes to recognize the signs and symptoms of concussion increases the likelihood of reporting the concussion to the appropriate personnel, which can decrease the risk of secondary consequences of concussion and prolonged recovery.[38,39]

In the last several decades, athletes have become stronger, faster, and smarter. These changes have been duplicated in technological advances of equipment, athletic rule changes, and even education about concussions and injuries that is based on research evidence. Public awareness and participation in sports demands more from health care professionals. While these advances occur in different sports, they share a common goal—to enhance the safety of all athletes.

Future Research and Innovations

Recent legislation requires education of all involved in athletics and medical care for athletes sustaining concussion. Education in concussion assessment and management would facilitate a thorough understanding of short- and long-term effects, recovery curves, and assessment techniques for concussive injuries. Currently, the legislation and concussion guidelines have been developed without a robust body of scientific evidence supporting these practices. Concussion research has begun to examine modifying factors to recovery, technology to aid in recovery, longitudinal studies of athletes participating in sport, among other research questions to obtain a greater understanding of concussions in athletes. Understanding all of these factors will improve the clinical care and treatment medical professionals and athletic trainers can provide following injury.

Researchers are continuing to investigate alternative assessment, management techniques, and comorbidities that may hinder recovery and present age-specific management techniques. Continued longitudinal studies that involve youth sports provide information on the course of the injury and long-term effects of concussion. Technological advances will help identify subtle changes in brain function, structure, and genetics that may affect susceptibility to concussions and modify the course of recovery. Furthermore, brain biopsies and autopsies of former athletes who sustained concussions might provide additional information.

The increase in suicide and violence from active and retired NFL players and military veterans returning home from active duty has provided evidence for additional theories regarding chronic traumatic encephalopathy (CTE), brain injury-related psychosis, and post-traumatic stress disorder (PTSD). The overarching diagnosis of concussion—which affects so many within different populations—has encouraged the need for additional resources to study and advance care for retired athletes, military suffering from PTSD, and adolescents with head injuries. These hypotheses have led many authorities to make recommendations regarding the safety of football. The most recent recommendation made by Dr. Robert Cantu during a television interview suggests delaying football participation until the child reaches 13 years of age. While this is an isolated opinion, researchers are striving to keep up with appropriate assessment and management techniques so clinicians can make athletics as safe as possible.

The focus of concussion research is changing from identifying and understanding the mechanism of the injury and clinical characteristics in adults, to examining adolescent and youth populations with a major focus on developing management plans and utilizing new technology to understand the underlying mechanisms and long-term sequelae following concussion.

There are many steps to be taken to completely understand this injury and the best clinical practices to return the concussed athlete back to his or her pre-injury state. It appears that the next logical steps will be influenced by technology and population needs inclusive of, but not limited to, athletes with comorbidities, population-based assessment tools, and intervention techniques to hasten recovery times. Other significant research foci in the future appear to trend toward the following:

- Critical time periods of injury and the effects of concussion during growth.

- Appropriate implementation of assessment tools: When should we test? What populations should we test? What should we use to test in each population?

- Management techniques to hasten recovery and prevent secondary injury.

- Long-term consequences of injury.

- The cumulative effect and dose response of subconcussive hits over an athletic career.

- Effectiveness of legislation and rule changes in athletics.

- Effectiveness of educational interventions across all populations.

- Neuroanatomical and neuropathological changes following injury.

- Biochemical markers to identify the presence of injury or recovery.

- Rehabilitation techniques across all populations to enhance recovery.

Clinicians are concerned that research has opened Pandora's box with concussion awareness. While this book focuses on sport-related concussion, concussions occur everywhere, from the playground to the battlefield. As clinicians, we strive to prevent injuries while trying to provide the best clinical care possible for everyone involved. Development of appropriate interventions and rehabilitation tools for those suffering from concussion, post-concussion syndrome, and CTE will not only support those currently in need, but future athletes, retirees, and weekend warriors. Opportunities to provide better treatment and management for concussion are expanding and are only hindered by the inability to come up with an idea. The future in this field is changing rapidly. Technological advances, increased funding for research, management options, and education for all involved in athletics is just the beginning.

Summary

- Concussions, unfortunately, are inherent in contact sports and there is limited evidence that any tool or technique can prevent the injury.

- There is some biomechanical evidence that helmet technology in football decreases the incidence of concussions.

- Education appears to increase the rate of reporting concussive signs and symptoms, but currently there is not enough evidence to determine decreases in catastrophic events from second impact syndrome or intracranial hematomas.

- Research presents conflicting results that mouthpieces and headgear in sports other than football reduce the risk of concussion.

- A strong research and clinical push is being made to ensure protective equipment has adequate evidence of a protective effect before clinicians support new technology use in athletics.

References

1. Hagel BE, Pless IB, Goulet C, et al. Effectiveness of helmets in skiers and snowboarders: case-control and case crossover study. *BMJ*. 2005;330:281-286.

2. Sulheim S, Holme I, Ekeland A, et al. Helmet use and risk of head injuries in alpine skiers and snowboarders. *JAMA*. 2006;295:919-924.

3. Mueller BA, Cummings P, Rivara FP, et al. Injuries of the head, face, and neck in relation to ski helmet use. *Epidemiology*. 2008;19:270-276.

4. Benson BW, Hamilton GM, Meeuwisse WH, McCrory P, Dvorak J. Is protective equipment useful in preventing concussion? A systematic review of the literature. *Br J Sports Med*. 2009;43(suppl 1):i56-i67.

5. McIntosh AS, McCrory P. Impact energy attenuation performance of football headgear. *Br J Sports Med*. 2000;34:337-341.

6. McIntosh A, McCrory P, Finch CF, et al. Does padded headgear prevent head injury in rugby union football? *Med Sci Sports Exerc*. 2009;41:306-313.

7. Pettersen JA. Does rugby headgear prevent concussion? Attitudes of Canadian players and coaches. *Br J Sports Med*. 2002;36:19-22.

8. Kemp SP, Hudson Z, Brooks JH, et al. The epidemiology of head injuries in English professional rugby union. *Clin J Sport Med*. 2008;18:227-234.

9. McIntosh A, McCrory P, Finch CF. Performance enhanced headgear: a scientific approach to the development of protective headgear. *Br J Sports Med*. 2004;38:46-49.

10. Marshall SW, Loomis DP, Waller AE, et al. Evaluation of protective equipment for prevention of injuries in rugby union. *Int J Epidemiol*. 2005;34(1):113-118.

11. Schwarz S. A case against helmets in lacrosse. *New York Times*. 2011. Retrieved at: http://www.nytimes.com/2011/02/17/sports/17lacrosse.html?pagewanted=all&_r=0. Accessed February 2, 2012.

12. Kerr I. Mouth guards for the prevention of injuries in contact sports. *Sports Med*. 1986;3:415-427.

13. McCrory P. Do mouthguards prevent concussion? *Br J Sports Med*. 2001;35:81-82.

14. Wisniewski J, Guskiewicz K, Trope M, et al. Incidence of cerebral concussions associated with type of mouthguard used in college football. *Dent Traumatol*. 2004;20:143-149.

15. Stenger J, Lawton E, Wright J, et al. Mouthguards: protection against shock to head, neck and teeth. *J Am Dent Assoc*. 1964;69:273-281.

16. Macleod S. Post concussion syndrome: the attraction of the psychological by the organic. *Med Hypotheses*. 2010;74:1033-1035.

17. Mainwaring L. Restoration of self: a model for the psychological response of athletes to severe knee injuries. *Canadian J Rehabil*. 1999;12:145-156.

18. Hickey J, Morris A, Carlson L, et al. The relation of mouth protectors to cranial pressure and deformation. *J Am Dent Assoc*. 1967;74:735-740.

19. Labella C, Smith B, Sigurdsson A. Effect of mouthguards on dental injuries and concussions in college basketball. *Med Sci Sports Exerc*. 2002;34:41-44.

20. Mihalik JP, McCaffrey MA, Rivera EM, et al. Effectiveness of mouthguards in reducing neurocognitive deficits following sports-related cerebral concussion. *Dent Traumatol*. 2007;23:14-20.

21. Newson PR, Tran DC, Cooke MS. The role of the mouthguard in the prevention of sports-related dental injuries: a review. *Int J Pediatric Dentistry*. 2001;11(6):396-404.

22. Finch C, Braham R, McIntosh A, McCrory P, Wolfe R. Should football players wear custom fitted mouthguards? Results from a group randomised controlled trial. *Inj Prev*. 2005;11(4):242-246.

23. Heck JF, Clark KS, Peterson PR, Torg JS, Weis MP. National athletic trainers' association position statement: head-down contact and spearing in tackle football. *J Athl Train*. 2004;39:101-111.

24. Torg JS. Epidemiology, biomechanics, and prevention of cervical spine trauma resulting from athletics and recreational activities. *Oper Tech Sports Med*. 1993;1:159.

25. Cantu RC, Mueller FO. Brain injury-related fatalities in American football, 1945-1999. *J Neurosurgery*. 2003;52(4):846-853.

26. Roux CE, Goedeke R, Visser GR, Van Zyl WA, Noakes TD. The epidemiology of schoolboy rugby injuries. *S Afr Med J*. 1987;71(7):307-313.

27. Stuart MJ, Smith AM, Malo-Ortiguera SA, et al. A comparison of facial protection and the incidence of head, neck, and facial injuries in Junior A hockey players. A function of individual playing time. *Am J Sports Med*. 2002;30:39-44.

28. Lemair M, Pearsall DJ. Evaluation of impact attenuation of facial protectors in ice hockey helmets. *Sports Eng*. 2007;10:65-74.

29. McCrory P, Meeuwisse W, Johnston K, et al. Consensus statement on concussion in sport, 3rd international conference on concussion in sport. Zurich 2008. *Clin J Sport Med*. 2009;19:185-200.

30. Aubry M, Cantu R, Dvorak J, et al. Summary and agreement statement of the First International Conference on Concussion in Sport, Vienna 2001: recommendations for the improvement of safety and health of athletes who may suffer concussive injuries. *Br J Sports Med*. 2002;36(1):6-10.

31. McCrory P, Johnston K, Meeuwisse W, et al. Summary and agreement statement of the 2nd International Conference on Concussion in Sport, Prague 2004. *Br J Sports Med*. 2005;39(4):196-204.

32. Guskiewicz KM, Bruce SL, Cantu R, et al. National Athletic Trainers' Association position statement: management of sport-related concussion. *J Athl Train*. 2004;39(3):280-297.

33. Powell JM, Ferraro JV, Dikman SS, Temkin NR, Bell KR. Accuracy of mild traumatic brain injury diagnosis. *Arch Phys Med Rehabil*. 2008;89(8):1550-1555.

34. Genuardi FJ, King WD. Inappropriate discharge instructions for youth athletes hospitalized for concussion. *Pediatrics*. 1995;95(2):216-218.

35. McCrea M, Hammeke T, Olsen G, Leo P, Guskiewicz K. Unreported concussion in high school football players: implications for prevention. *Clin J Sport Med*. 2004;14(1):13-17.

36. Valovich McLeod TC, Bay RC, Heil J, McVeigh SD. Identification of sport and recreational activity concussion history through the pre-participation screening and a symptom survey in young athletes. *Clin J Sport Med*. 2008;18:235-240.

37. Kaut KP, DePompei R, Kerr J, Congeni J. Reports of head injury and symptoms knowledge among college athletes: implications for assessment and educational intervention. *Clin J Sports Med*. 2003;13(4):213-221.

38. Bramley HP, Patrick K, Lehman E, Silvis M. High school soccer players with concussion education are more likely to notify their coach of a suspected concussion. *Clin Pediatr*. 2012;51(4):332-336.

39. Sye G, Sullivan SJ, McCrory P. High school rugby players' understanding of concussion and return to play guidelines. *Br J Sports Med*. 2006;40:1003-1005.

SUGGESTED READINGS

Concussion Position Statements

- National Athletic Trainers' Association Position Statement: Management of Sport-related Concussion. Available at: http://www.nata.org/sites/default/files/MgmtOfSportRelatedConcussion.pdf

- Consensus statement on concussion in sport—Summary and Agreement Statements of the First International Conference on Concussion in Sport. Available at: http://bjsportmed.com/content/36/1/6.full.pdf

- Consensus statement on concussion in sport—Summary and Agreement Statements of the Second International Conference on Concussion in Sport. *J Clinical Neuroscience*. Available at: http://www.amssm.org/Content/pdf20files/2012_ConcussionPositionStmt.pdf

- Consensus statement on concussion in sport—Summary and Agreement Statements of the Third International Conference on Concussion in Sport. *Br J Sports Medicine*. Available at: http://bjsportmed.com/content/39/4/196.full.pdf

- Consensus statement on concussion in sport—Summary and Agreement Statements of the Fourth International Conference on Concussion in Sport. Available at: http://journals.lww.com/acsm-msse/Fulltext/2011/12000/Concussion__Mild_Traumatic_Brain_Injury__and_the.24.aspx#

Within the Fourth International Conference, the following additional tools were proposed and created:

  ▷ The new tools update the current SCAT 2. Available at: http://bjsm.bmj.com/content/47/5/259.full.pdf

  ▷ Provide an applicable sideline tool for adolescents and children. Available at: http://bjsm.bmj.com/content/47/5/263.full.pdf

  ▷ Provide a pocket reference card for ease of use and clinical care. Available at: http://bjsm.bmj.com/content/47/5/267.full.pdf

- American Medical Society for Sports Medicine (AMSSM): Concussion in Sport. Available at: http://www.amssm.org/Content/pdf%20files/2012_ConcussionPositionStmt.pdf

- Concussion (Mild Traumatic Brain Injury) and the Team Physician: A Consensus Statement. Available at: http://journals.lww.com/acsm-msse/Fulltext/2011/12000/Concussion__Mild_Traumatic_Brain_Injury__and_the.24.aspx

- American Academy of Neurology (AAN) Position Statement on Sports Concussion. Available at: http://www.aan.com/globals/axon/assets/7913.pdf

- American Academy of Pediatrics (AAP)- Sport-related Concussion in Children and Adolescents. Available at: http://pediatrics.aappublications.org/content/126/3/597.full.pdf

Internet Resources

Centers for Disease Control

The Centers for Disease Control (CDC) provides publicly available information for a significant amount of diseases and conditions. Within the last decade, alongside the National Institute of Injury Prevention and Control, the CDC has focused on providing more information regarding concussion. For more information visit www.cdc.gov/concussion

The CDC started the Heads Up program in 2005 and continues to update and incorporate new research, educational interventions and multiple populations such as health care providers, administrators, coaches, parents, and athletes. There are numerous versions of educational material from the Center for Disease control. For more information visit http://www.cdc.gov/concussion/HeadsUp/schools.html

To enhance the educational portion of the program, free online training has been available since 2011 through the CDC Web site. This training discusses the prominent features of concussion, prevention techniques and return to participation and school recommendations. After completion of the course, there is a printable certificate. For more information visit http://www.cdc.gov/concussion/headsup/online_training

Reduce, Educate, Accommodate, and Pace Program

The Reduce, Educate, Accommodate, and Pace (REAP) program was developed in Colorado and emphasizes the team approach to concussion management in a school setting. For more information visit http://cokidswithbraininjury.com/mild-tbi-concussion-info

National Federation of High School Associations

There is extensive information and educational opportunities for high school athletics, "Concussion in Sports—What You Need to Know." For more information visit http://www.nfhslearn.com/electiveDetail. aspx?courseID=15000

Government Accountability Office on Head Injury

The Government Accountability Office (GAO) has been charged with evaluation of youth concussion databases and prevention practices across the nation. For more information visit www.gao.gov

In 2011, the GAO was asked to testify in front of the Committee on Education and Labor in the House of Representatives on "Concussion in High School Sports: Overall Estimate of Occurrence Is Not Available, but Key State Laws and Nationwide Guidelines Address Injury Management." For more information visit: http://www.gao.gov/assets/130/124717.pdf

Online Concussion Education Training

ThinkFirst Concussion Education Online. Available at: http://concussioneducation.ca/

National Federation of High School Concussion in Sport Online Course. Available at: http://www.nfhslearn.com/

Athletic Concussion Training using Interactive Video Education (ACTive): Athletic Concussion Training: http://brain101.orcasinc.com/4000/

Sport Concussion Library

The sport concussion library was started in 2011 by Paul Echlin and provides educational information for parents, coaches, and educational support staff. This Web site is easy to navigate for all involved in concussion education and contains up-to-date information for all involved. For more information visit http://www.sportconcussionlibrary.com

Reference Books

Carroll L, Rosner D. *The Concussion Crisis: Anatomy of a Silent Epidemic*. New York, NY: Simon & Schuster; 2011

Humm JL, Kozlowski DA, James DC, Gotts JE, Schallert T. Use-dependent exacerbation of brain damage occurs during an early post-lesion vulnerable period. *Brain Res*. 1998;783(2):286-292.

Lovell, M, ed. *Traumatic Brain Injury in Sports: An International Neuropsychological Perspective*. Exton, PA: Swets & Zeitlinger; 2004.

Meehan, WP. *Kids, Sports, and Concussion: A Guide for Coaches and Parents.* Santa Barbara, CA: Praeger; 2011.

Ruben J. Echemendia, ed. *Sports Neuropsychology: Assessment and Management of Traumatic Brain Injury.* New York, NY: Guilford Press; 2006.

Slobounov S, Seastianelli W, eds. *Foundations of Sport-Related Brain Injuries.* Boston, MA: Springer; 2010.

INDEX

accommodation, after concussion, 99–105
age
    in concussion incidence, 5–6
    related to recovery, 82
alpha II spectrin breakdown proteins, 67
al-Razi, Abu Bakr Muhammad ibn Zakariya, 1
American Academy of Neurology, grading scale, 60
Americans with Disabilities Act, 100
amitriptyline, 80
anatomic considerations, 7–9
animal models, metabolic cascade, 11–12
ApoE-4 protein, 67

balance, evaluation, 54–56, 63–65
Balance Error Scoring System (BESS), 56–57
baseline testing, 36–38
    individualized baseline testing, 36–37
    mass baseline testing, 37–38
brain decade, 2
brainstem, anatomy, 7–8

calcium, in pathophysiology, 12
Cantu grading scale, 60
Centers for Disease Control
    Heads Up program, 2–3, 128
    information resources, 128–129
centripetal theory of injury, 9–10
cerebellum, anatomy, 9
cerebrovascular disease, stroke, 27–28
cerebrum, anatomy, 8
chronic traumatic encephalopathy, 122–123
Clinical reaction time measure, 66
Clinical Test of Sensory Interaction of Balance, 65
cognitive function, assessment, 50, 52, 60–61
cognitive rest, 78–79
cognitive symptoms, 39
Colorado grading scale, 60
comminuted skull fractures, 24

commotio cerebri, 1–2
computed tomography, 58
concussion
    definition, 3–5
    previous history, 83–84
Concussion in Sport Group guidelines, for return to participation, 94–98
Congress of Neurological Surgeons, Head Injury Nomenclature, 4
consensus statements, 127–128
contrecoup injury, 9
costs, of sport-related concussions, 3
coup injury, 9
coup/contrecoup model, 9
cranial nerves, evaluation, 50–51

decerebrate posturing, 45
decorticate posturing, 45
depressed skull fractures, 24
depression, 85
    spreading, 12
dermatomes, evaluation, 48
diencephalon, anatomy, 8
differential diagnoses, 19–34
docosahexaenoic acid, 80

education, for concussion prevention, 121–122, 129
Edwin Smith Papyrus, 1
effort, in test sessions, 85–86
employment, return to, 99–105
environmental influences, on recovery, 84–85
epidemiology
    age factors, 5–6
    gender differences, 6
    mortality statistics, 5
    player position, 6–7
    self-reporting, 6–7
epidural hematomas, 20–21
epilepsy, 25–26
evaluation, 35–75
    balance, 54–56, 63–65
    baseline testing, 36–38
    clinical tools, 65–68

in concussion management plan, 111, 114
Glasgow Coma Scale, 56–58
grading scales, 59–60
imaging, 58–59
King-Devick test, 56
neurocognitive assessment, 60–61
neurologic examination, 47–51
palpation, 47
physical examination, 41–46
self-reported symptoms, 38–41
sideline balance testing, 54–56
sideline cognitive assessment, 50, 52
Sport Concussion Assessment Tool, 53–54
Sport Concussion Office Assessment Tool, 61–63
Standardized Assessment of Concussion tool, 52–53
executive function, 84
exercise
in management program, 83
rest from, 78–79, 83
exertional heat illness, 28–29
exhaustion, heat, 28–29
eye
inspection, 45–46
response in Glasgow Coma Scale, 57

Family Medical Leave Act, 103
federal legislation, 107–108, 122
flexion contracture, 45
force platforms, for balance testing, 64
fractures, skull, 24–25
functional magnetic resonance imaging, 58–59

gender, in concussion incidence, 6
generalized seizure disorder, 25–26
genetic markers, for concussion assessment, 66–68
Glasgow Coma Scale, 56–58
glucose abnormalities, 12
glutamate, in pathophysiology, 11
Government Accountability Office, 129
Graded Symptom Checklist, 40
Graded Symptom Scale, 40
grading scales, 59–60

Head Injury Scale, 40
headers, 11
headgear, 2, 119–120
Heads Up program, 2–3, 128
heat illness, exertional, 28–29
helmets, 2, 119–120
hematomas, 20–22
hemorrhagic stroke, 27–28
Hippocratic Corpus, 1
historical perspective, 1–3
history, in physical examination, 41, 43–44
hyperbaric oxygen therapy, 80–81

imaging, 58–59
Individual education program, 100–104
Individuals with Disabilities Education Act, 100–104
incidence, *see* epidemiology
information resources, 127–130
inspection, visual, 44–46
International Conference on Concussion in Sport
    concussion definition, 4–5
    consensus statement, 127–128
internet resources, 128–129
ischemic stroke, 27–28

King-Devick test, 56
Kirkland, Thomas, 2

Lanfrancus, Guido, 1–2
learning disabilities, recovery, 84
legal precedent, 107–118
    concussion management plan development, 110–117
    legislation, 107–108, 122
    National Collegiate Athletic Association recommendations, 109–110
    National Federation of State High School Associations (NFHS), 3,
        108-109, 117, 120
legislation, federal and state, 107–108, 122
library, for sport concussion, 129
linear skull fractures, 24
loss of consciousness, 43–44
lower quarter screens, 48–50

Maddocks questions, 52
magnetic resonance imaging, 58–59
management, of concussion
    guidelines, 77–81
    improper, 83
    plan, 110–117
Max's Law, 107
mechanism of injury, 9–12
medications, for concussion symptoms, 79–81
memory testing, 52
metabolic cascade, 11–12
Military Acute Concussion Evaluation, 56
motor response, in Glasgow Coma Scale, 57
mouth guards, 120
myotomes, evaluation, 49

National Athletic Trainers' Association protocol, 107
National Collegiate Athletic Association recommendations, 109–110, 120
National Federation of State High School Associations
    guidelines, 108–109, 120
    information resources, 129
National Football League mandates, 109, 121
NeuroCom Smart Balance Master, 64
neurologic examination, 47–50
nicotinamide, 80
Nintendo Wii Fit Balance Board, 65–66
nomenclature, 3–4
nystagmus, 48

oculomotor function, evaluation, 56
omega-3 fatty acids, 80
orientation, assessment, 52
over-stimulation, avoidance, 102
oxygen therapy, hyperbaric, 80–81

palpation, in physical examination, 47
participation, return to, 93–98
pharmacologic treatment, 79–81
physical activity, rest from, 78–79
physical examination, 41–46
physical therapy, 81
physiologic mechanism, for concussion, 11–12

physiological symptoms, 39
player position, in concussion incidence, 6–7
pointing task, for balance evaluation, 66
position statements, concussion, 127–128
positron emission tomography, 58–59
Post-Concussion Scale, 40–42
post-concussion syndrome, 31–32
postural stability, evaluation, 54–56, 63–65
posturing, 45
potassium, in pathophysiology, 11–12
prevention, 119–126
    education, 121–122
    headgear, 2, 119–120
    mouth guards, 120
    research, 122–124
    rule changes, 120–121
Protecting Student-Athletes from Concussion Acts of 2011 and 2012, 107
protective equipment, 119–121
punch-drunk syndrome, 2
pupils
    inspection, 46
    reaction to light, 47

REAP (Reduce, Educate, Accommodate and Pace) program, 114, 128
recovery, from concussion
    barriers, 77–78
    factors influencing, 81–85
    prognosis, 78
    stages, 77
reflexes, evaluation, 49–50
repeated subconcussive forces, 10–11
research, 122–124
rest, 78–79
return
    to participation, 93–98
    to school and work, 99–105
Rivermead Post-Concussion Symptom Questionnaire, 40
Romberg test, 54–55
rotational forces, 9–10
rules, for injury protection, 120–121

Safety of School Sports—Concussions, 107
S100B protein, 67
school, return to, 99–105
second impact syndrome, 23–24
seizures, 25–26
self-reported symptoms, 38–41
serial 7s, in cognitive assessment, 50
sideline assessments
    balance, 54–56
    cognitive, 50, 52
single-photon emission computed tomography, 58–59
skull, fracture, 24–25
Smith, Edwin, 1
social factors, in recovery, 85
socioeconomic status, recovery, 84–85
sodium-potassium pump, in pathophysiology, 11–12
somatic symptoms, 39
spectrin breakdown proteins, 67
Sport Concussion Assessment Tool, 53–54
sport concussion library, 129
Sport Concussion Office Assessment Tool, 61–63
spreading depression, 12
Standardized Assessment of Concussion tool, 52–53
state legislation, 107–108, 122
stroke
    in cerebrovascular disease, 27–28
    heat, 28–29
subconcussive forces, repeated, 10–11
subdural hematomas, 21–22
suicide, in concussed athletes, 122
symptoms, self-reported, 38–41

tanking, 85–86
three-word recall test, 52
treatment, of concussion
    guidelines, 77–81
    improper, 83
    plan, 110–117

upper quarter screens, 48–50

verbal response, in Glasgow Coma Scale, 57
violent behavior, in concussed athletes, 122
vision, evaluation, 46
visual inspection, 44–46
Visuomotor Pointing Test, 66
vitamin B3, 80

Wii Fit Balance Board, 65–66
work, return to, 99–105

x-rays, 58

Zachery Lystedt law, 3, 107, 109
Zurich guidelines, for return to participation, 94–98

Printed in the United States
by Baker & Taylor Publisher Services